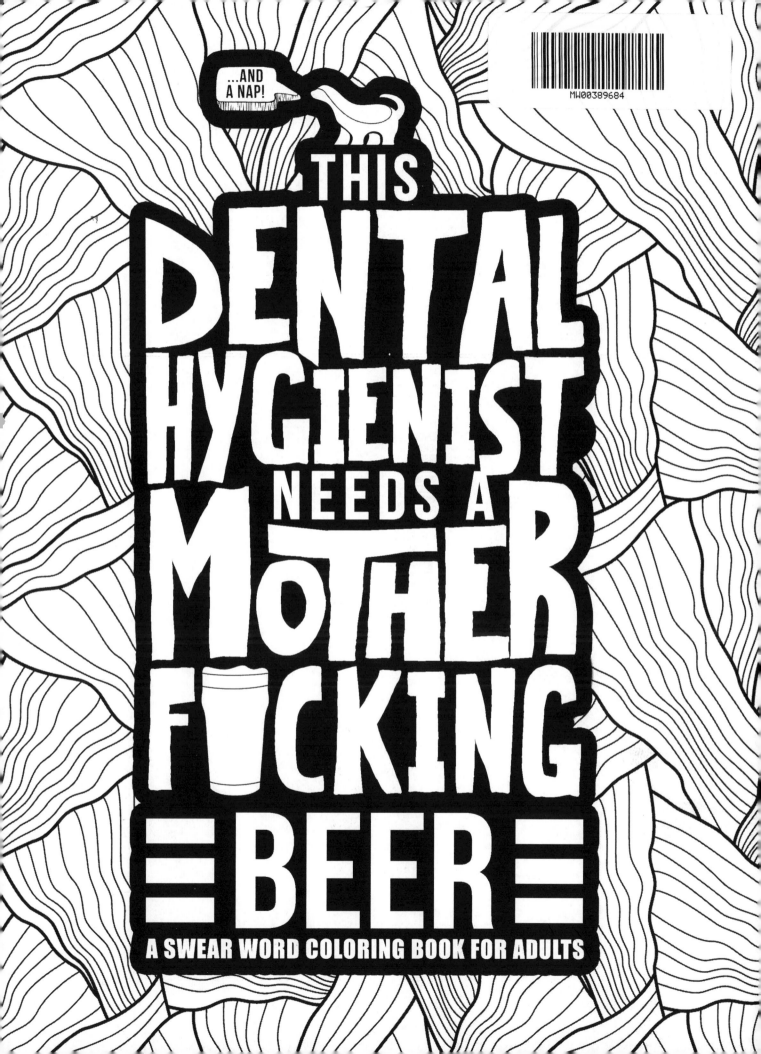

Want free goodies?
Email us at freebies@honeybadgercoloring.com

@honeybadgercoloring

Honey Badger Coloring

Shop our other books at
www.honeybadgercoloring.com

Wholesale distribution through Ingram Content Group
www.ingramcontent.com/publishers/distribution/wholesale

For questions and customer service, email us at
support@honeybadgercoloring.com

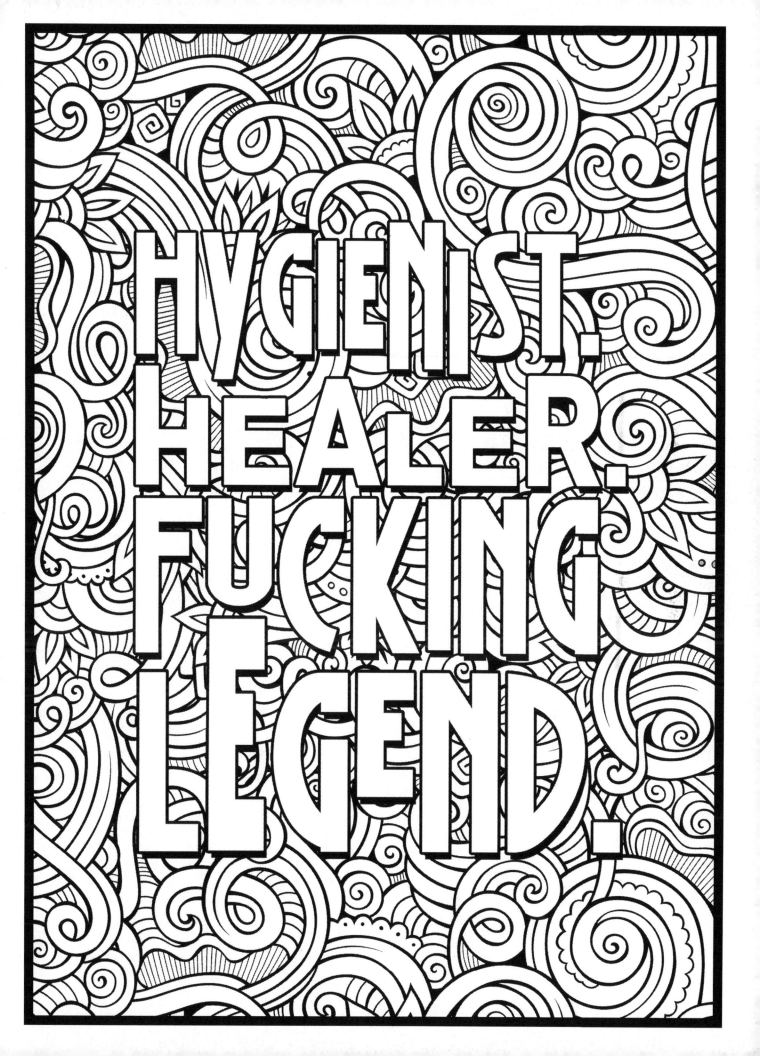

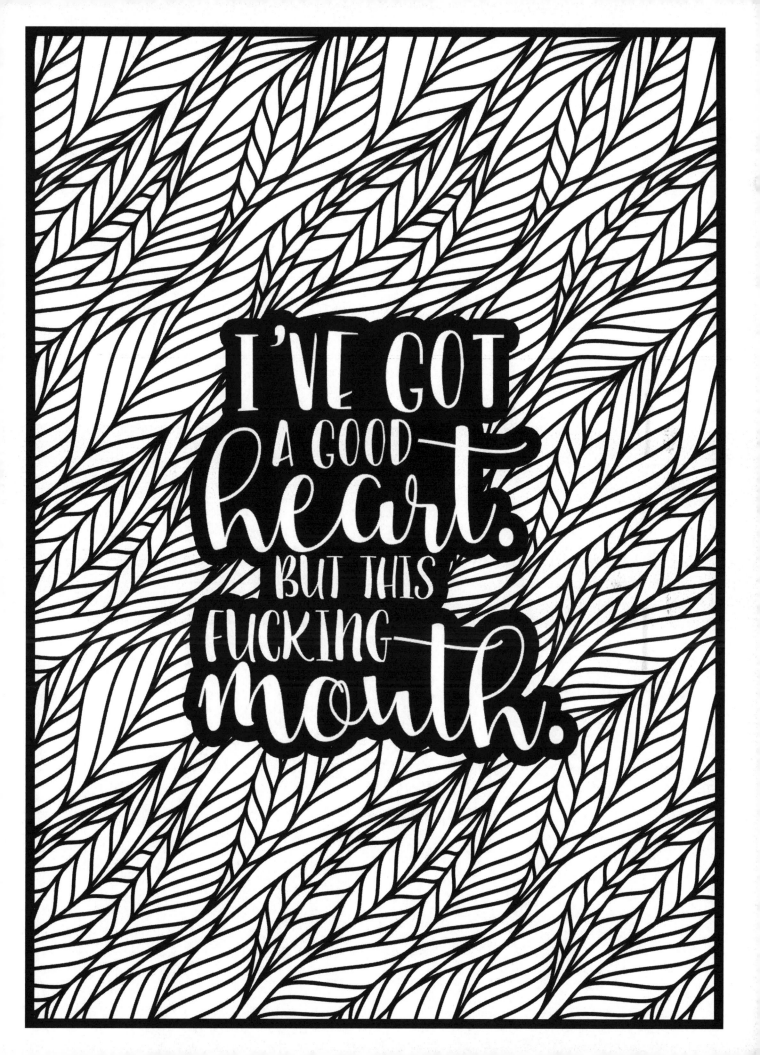

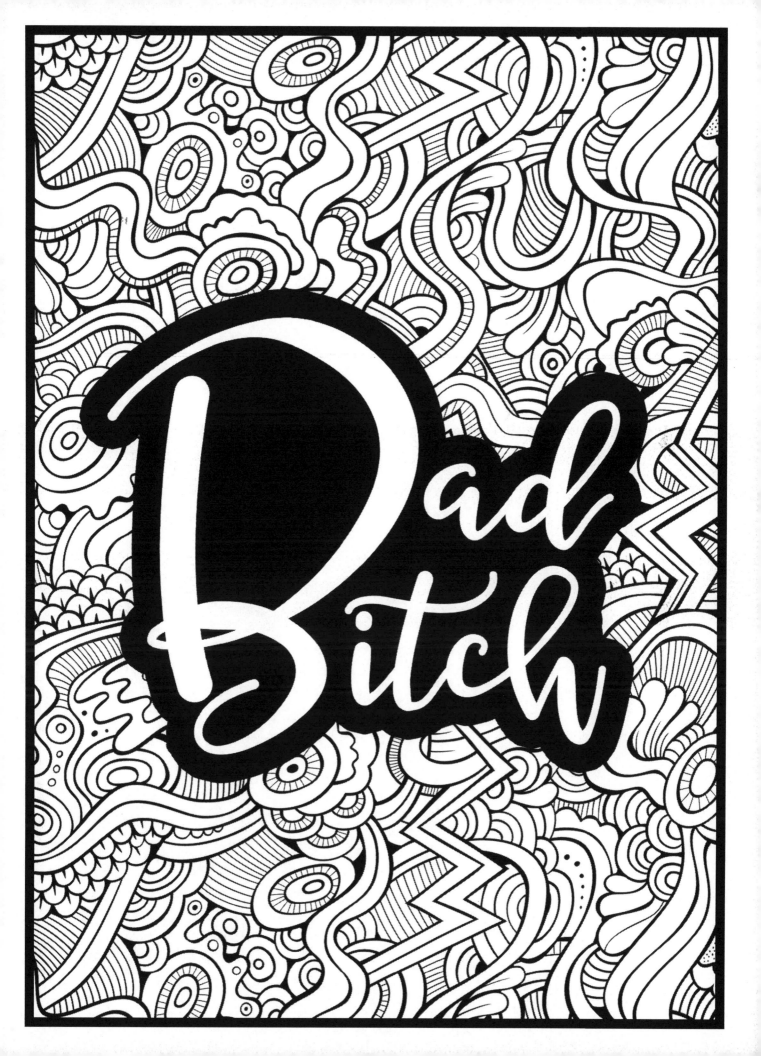

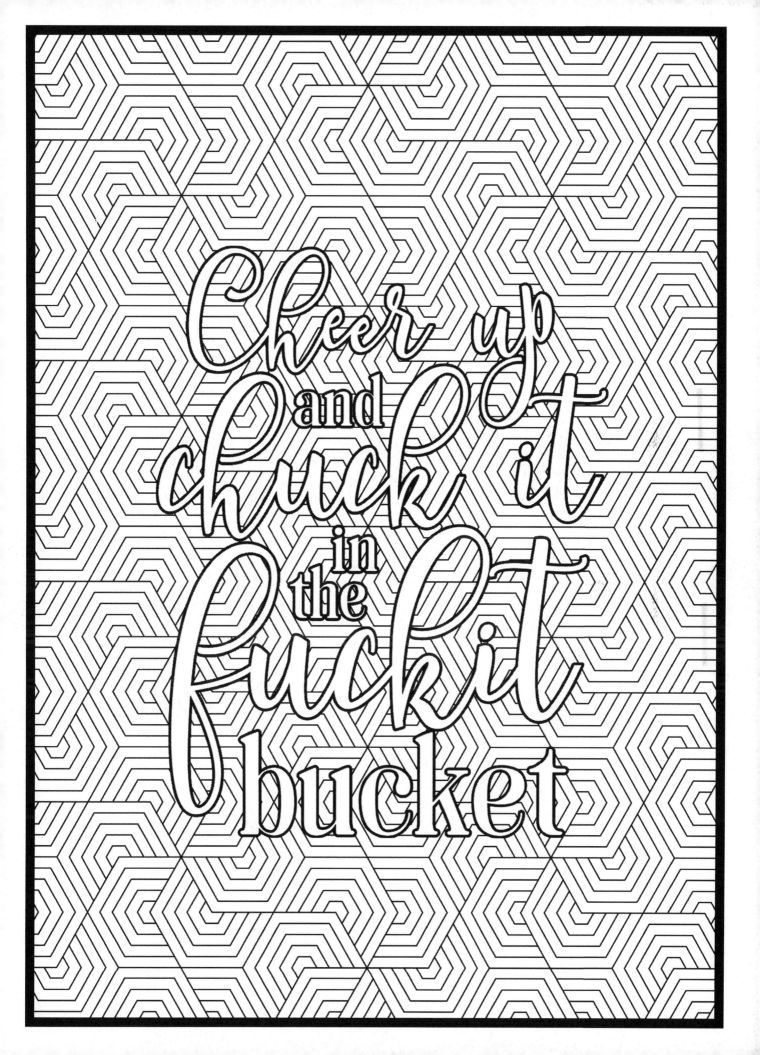

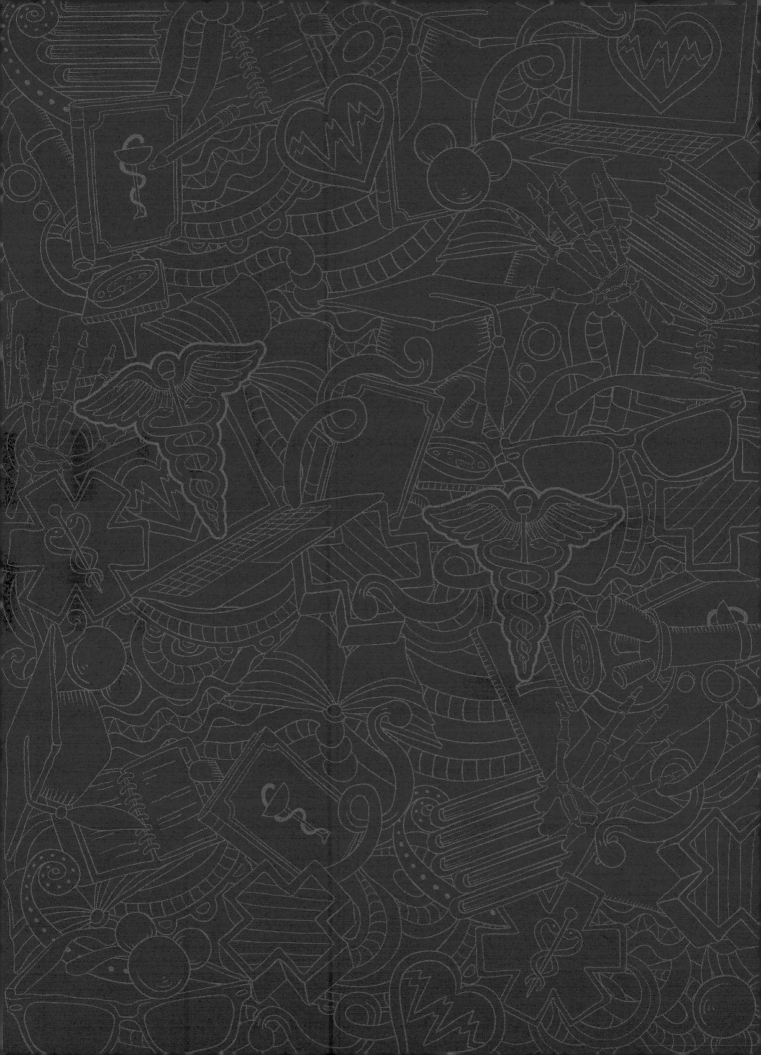

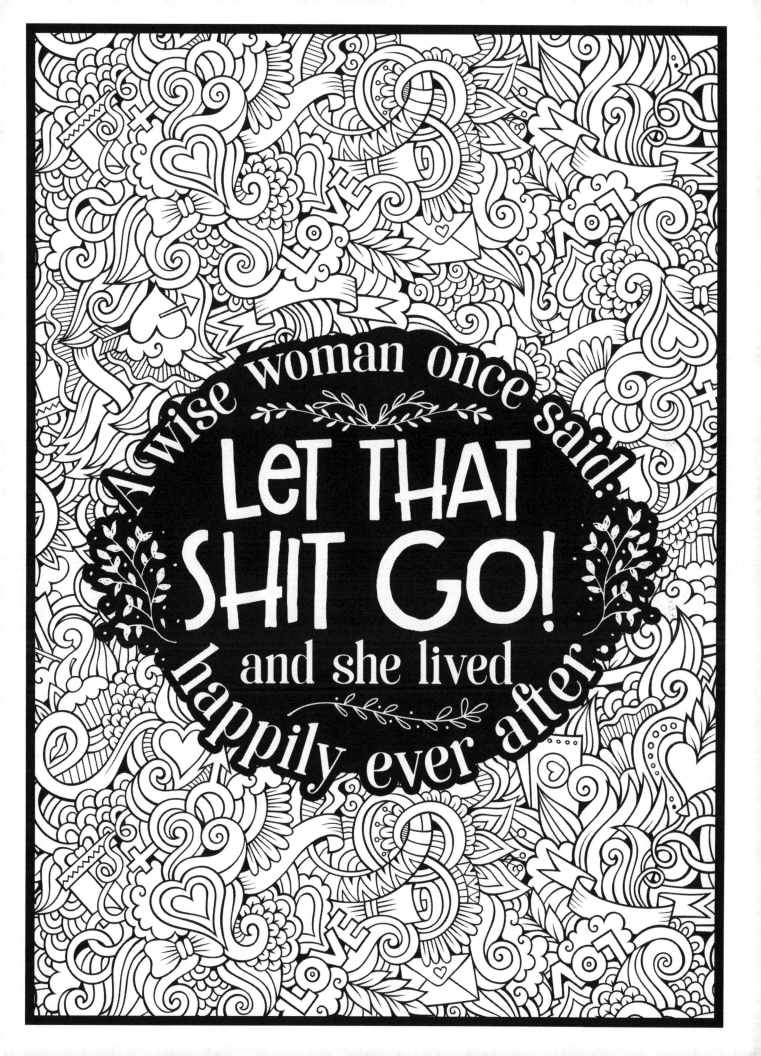

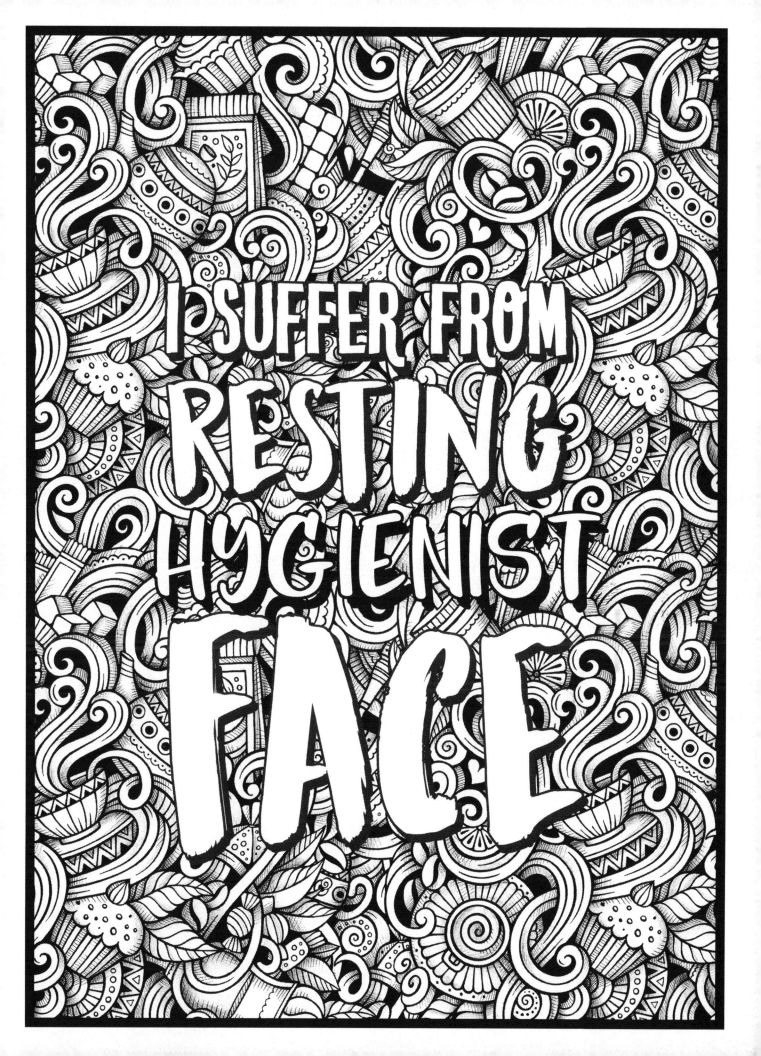

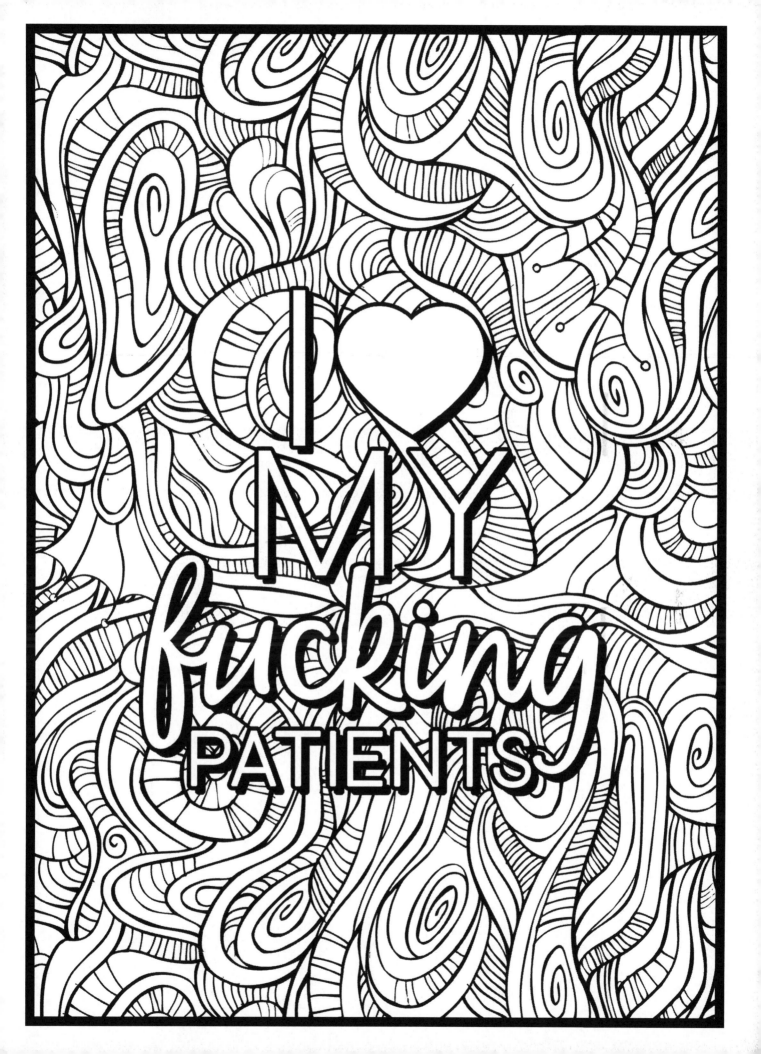

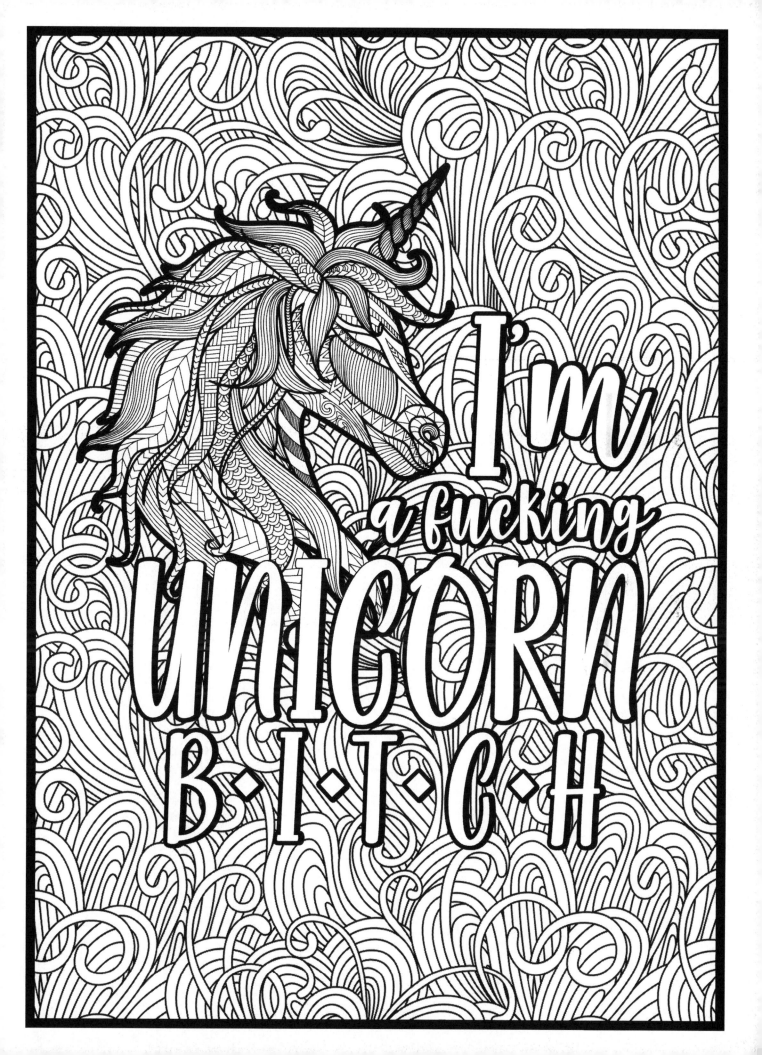

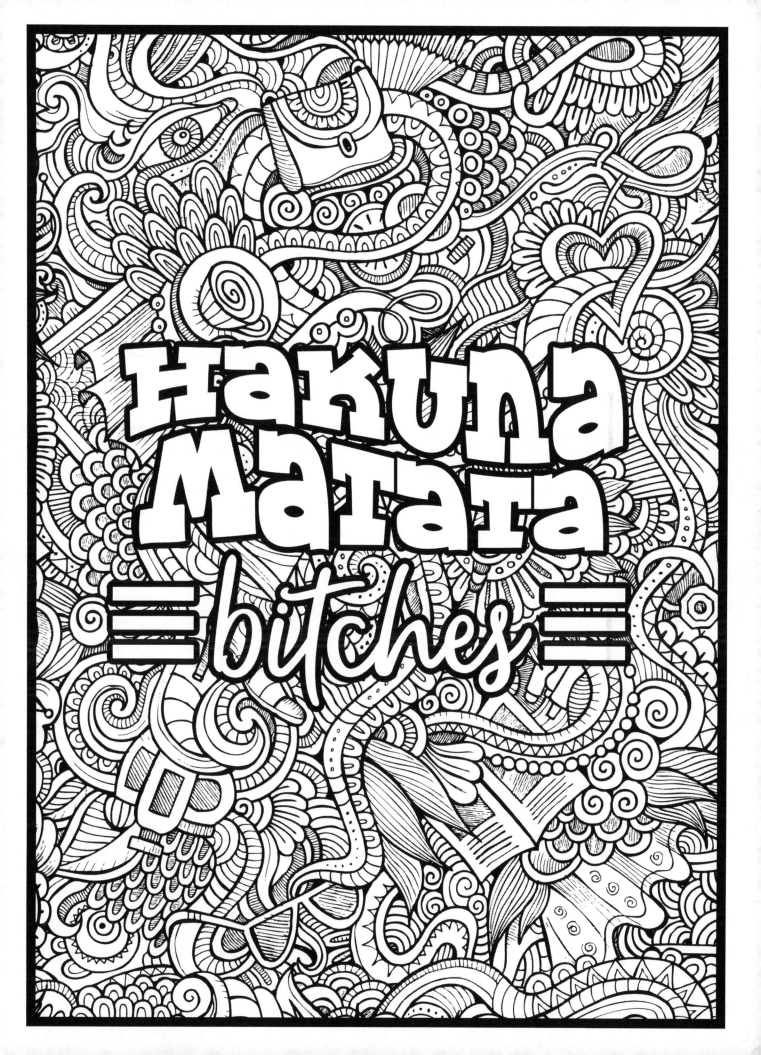

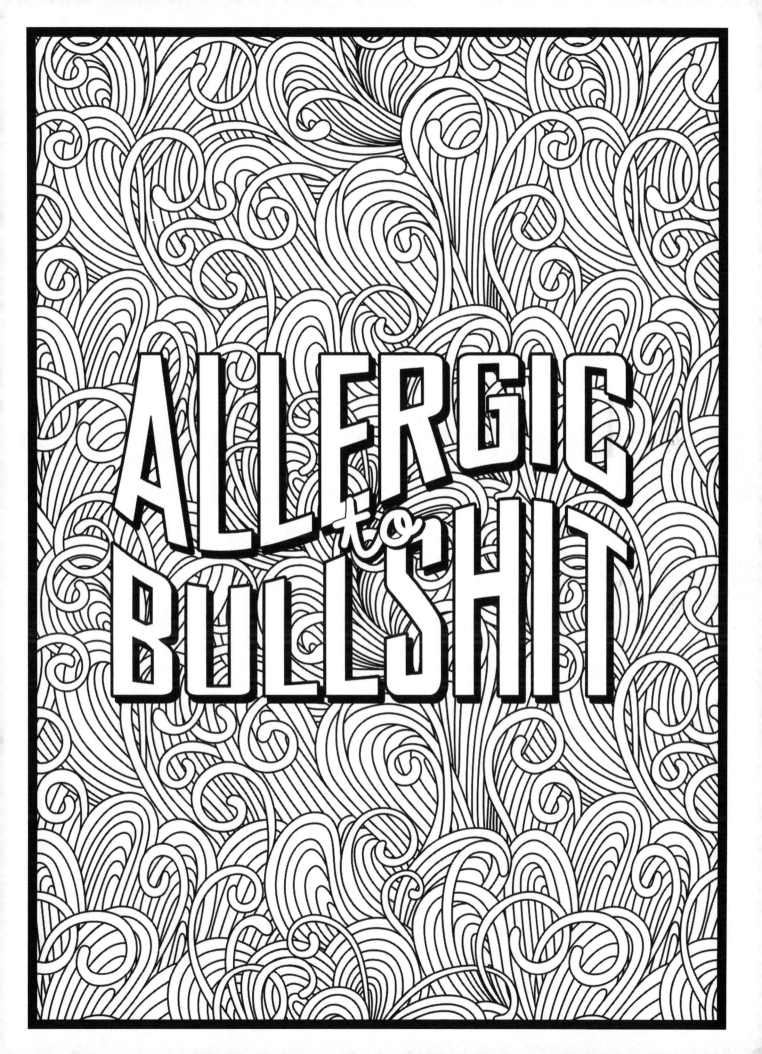

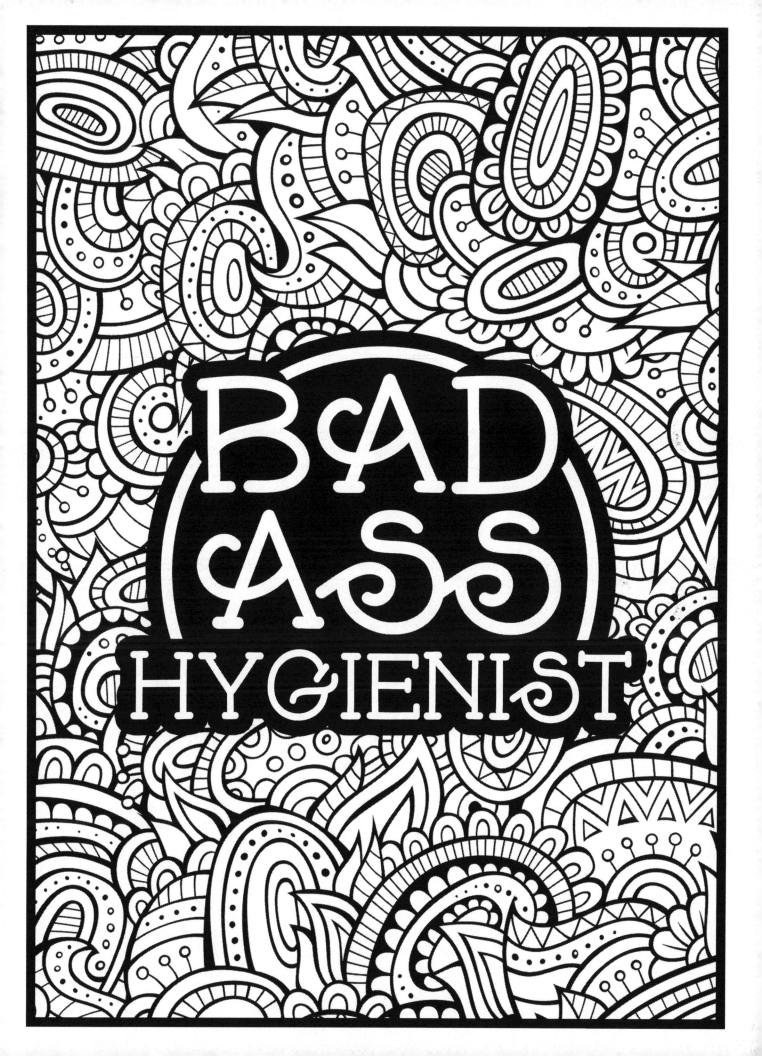

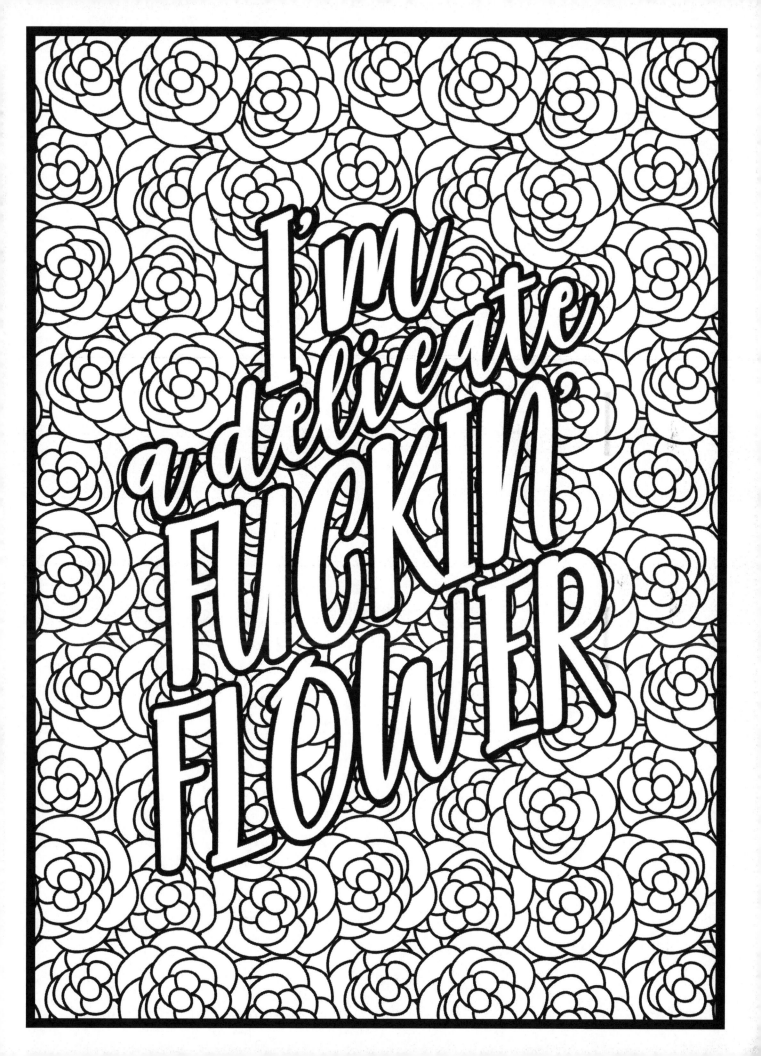

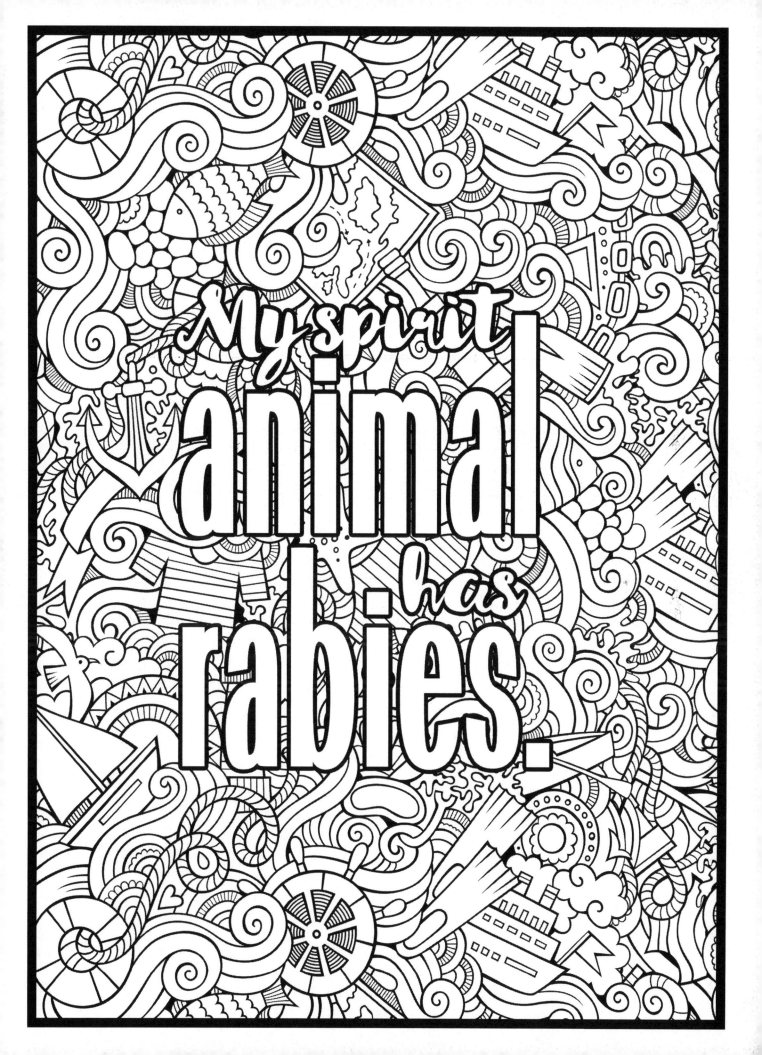

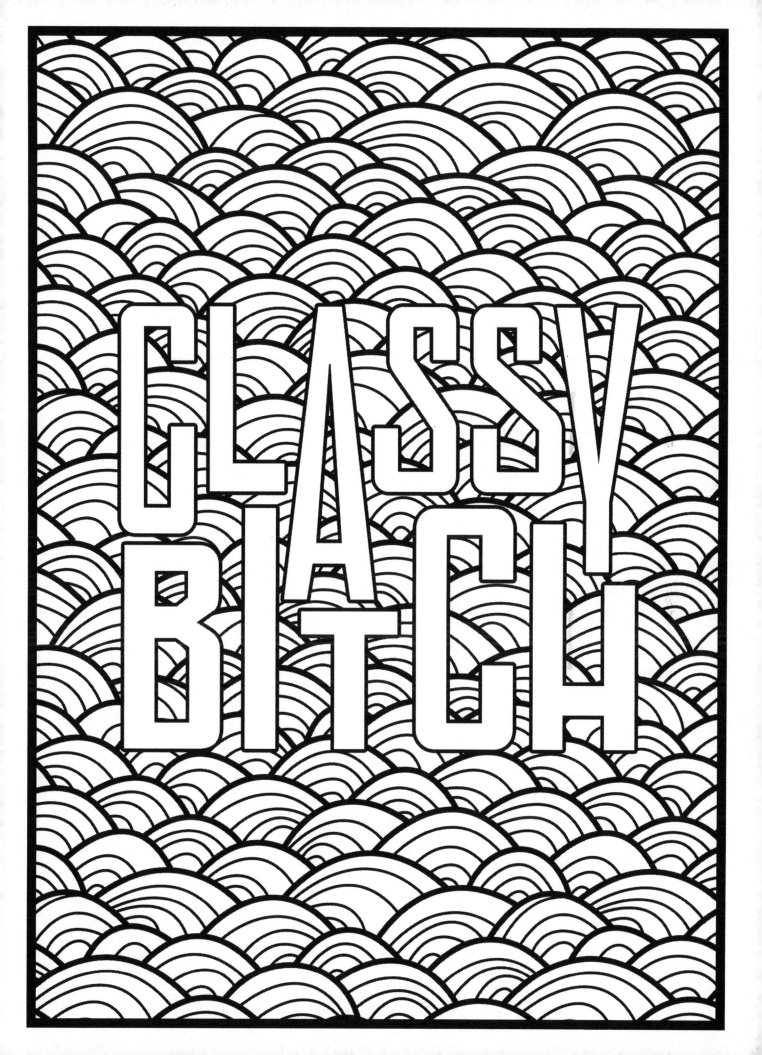

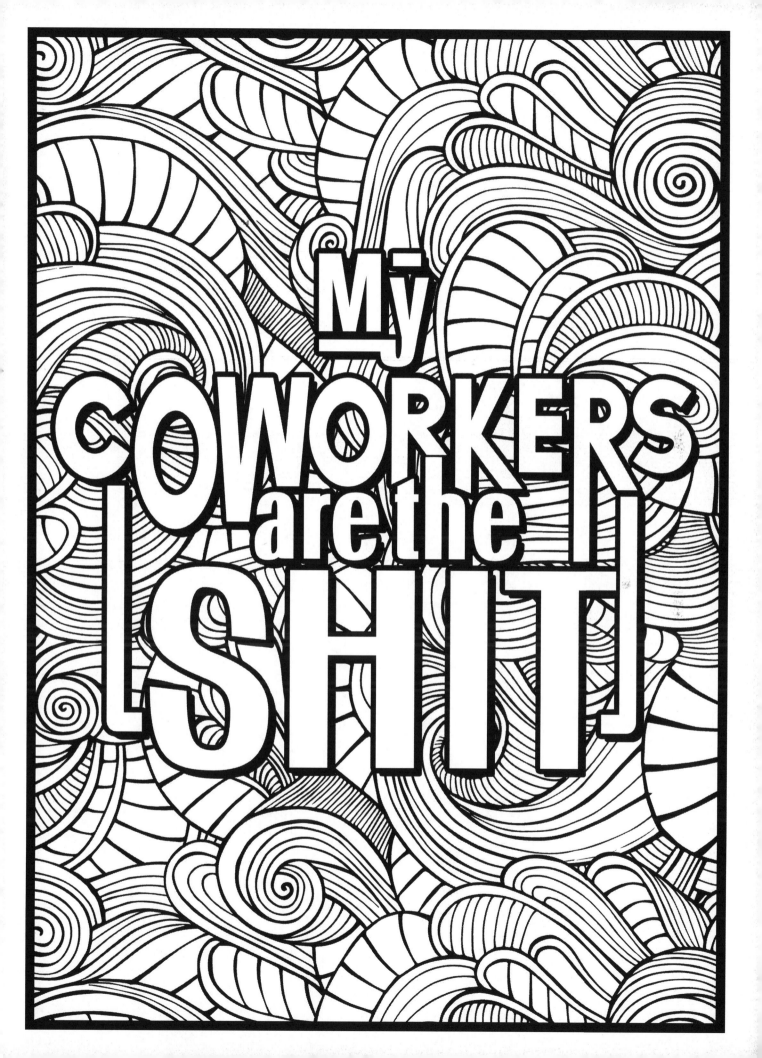

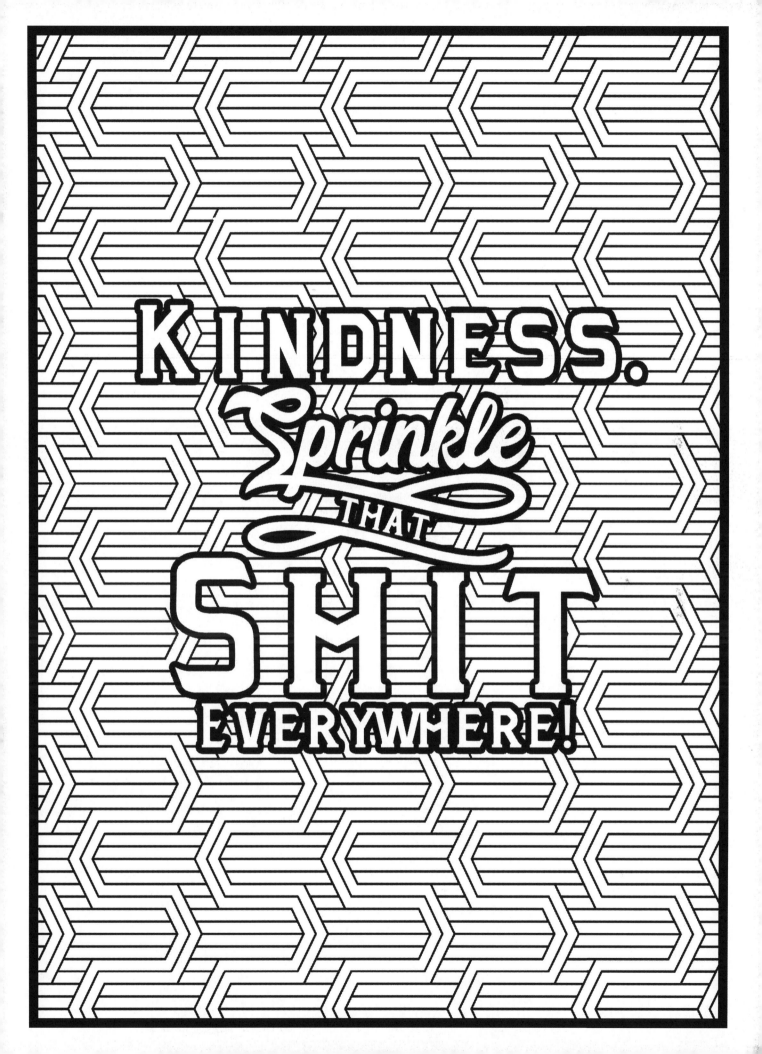

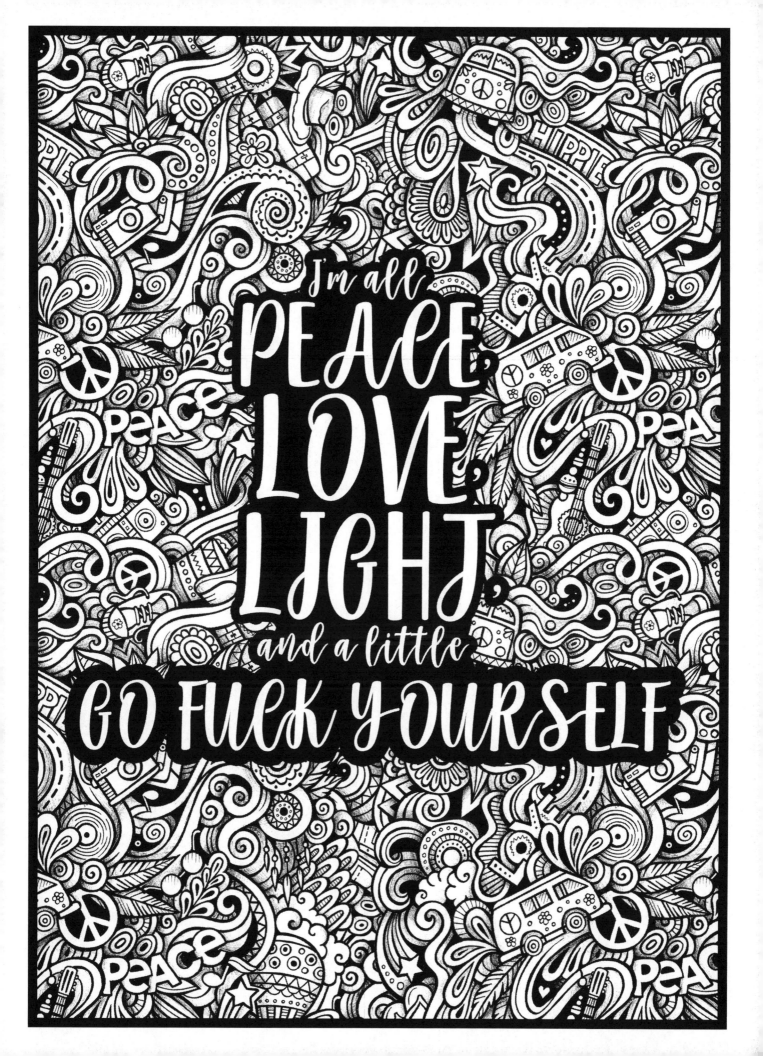

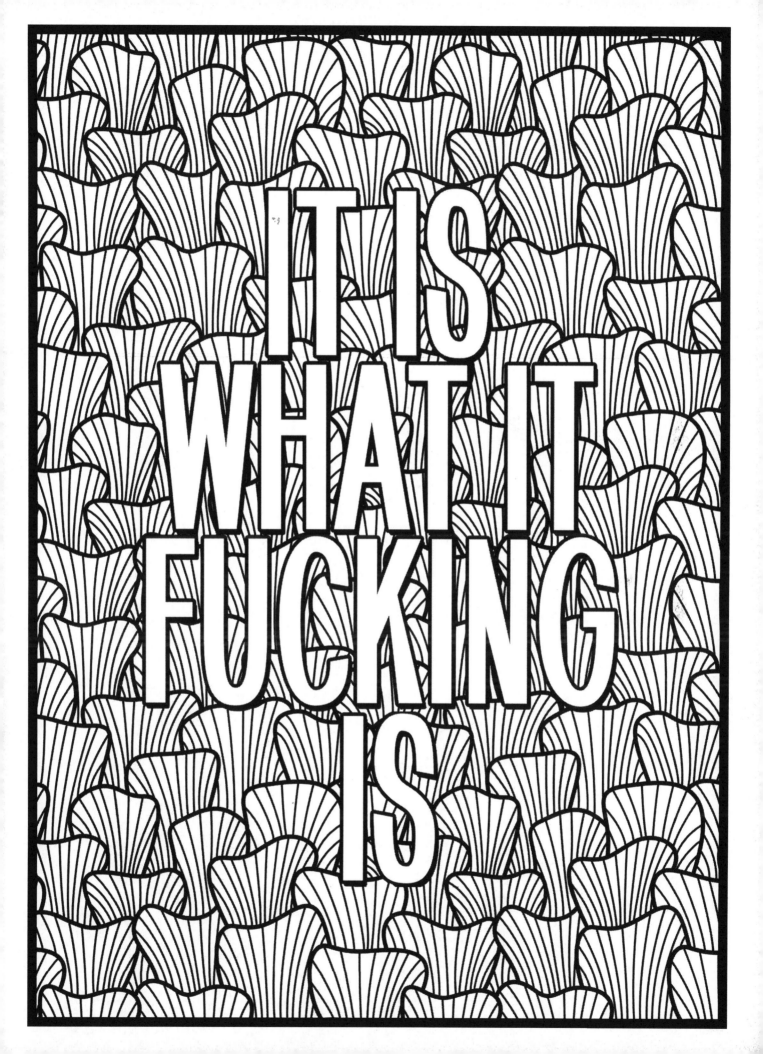

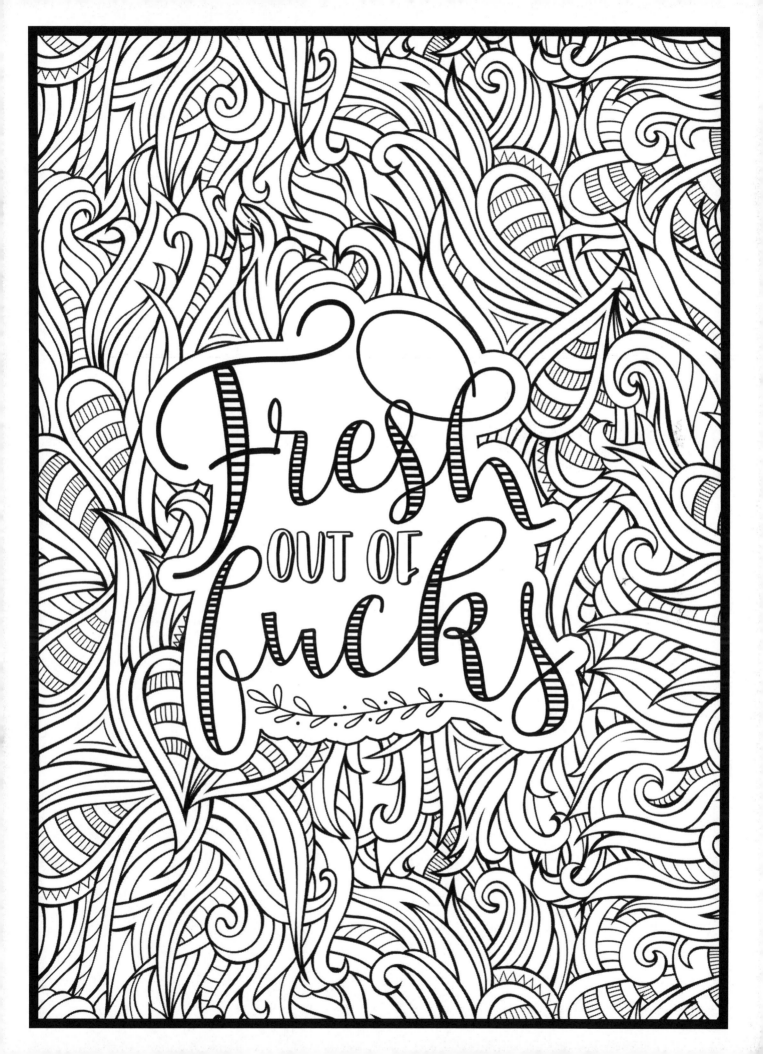

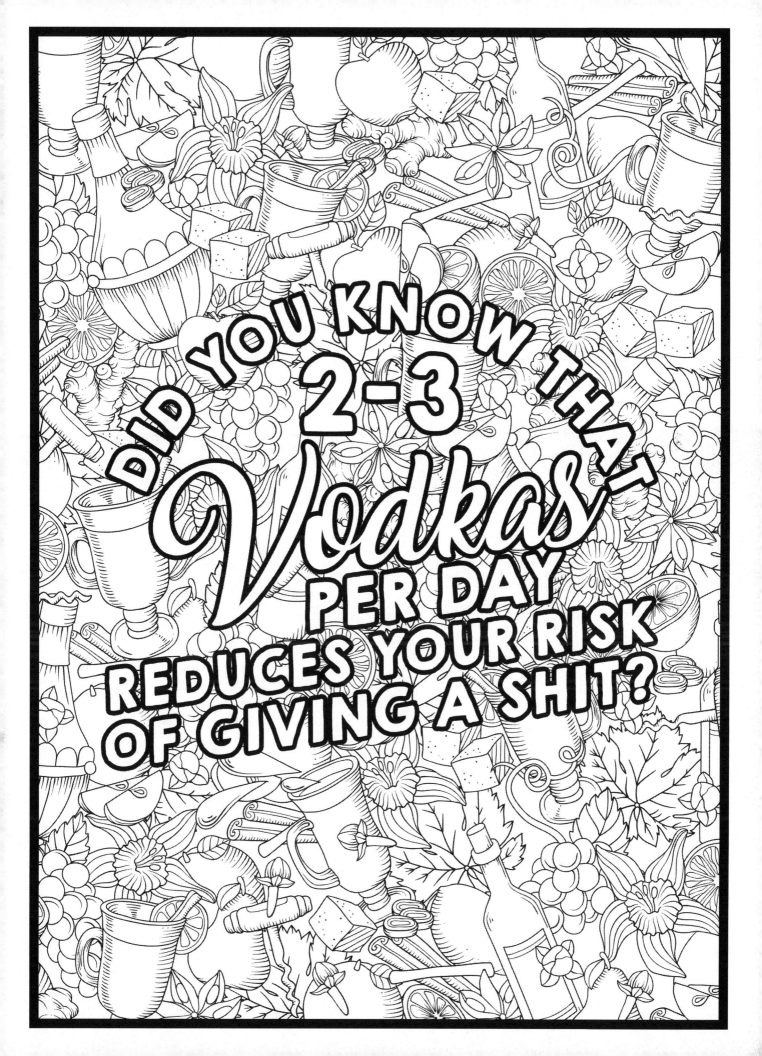

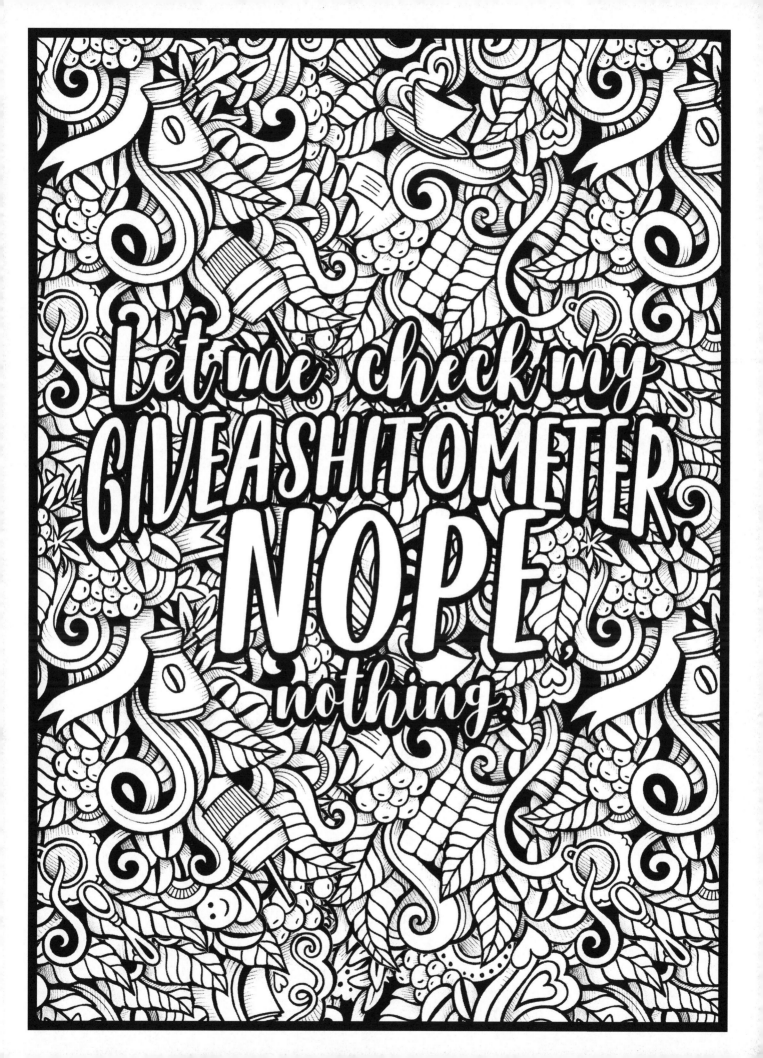

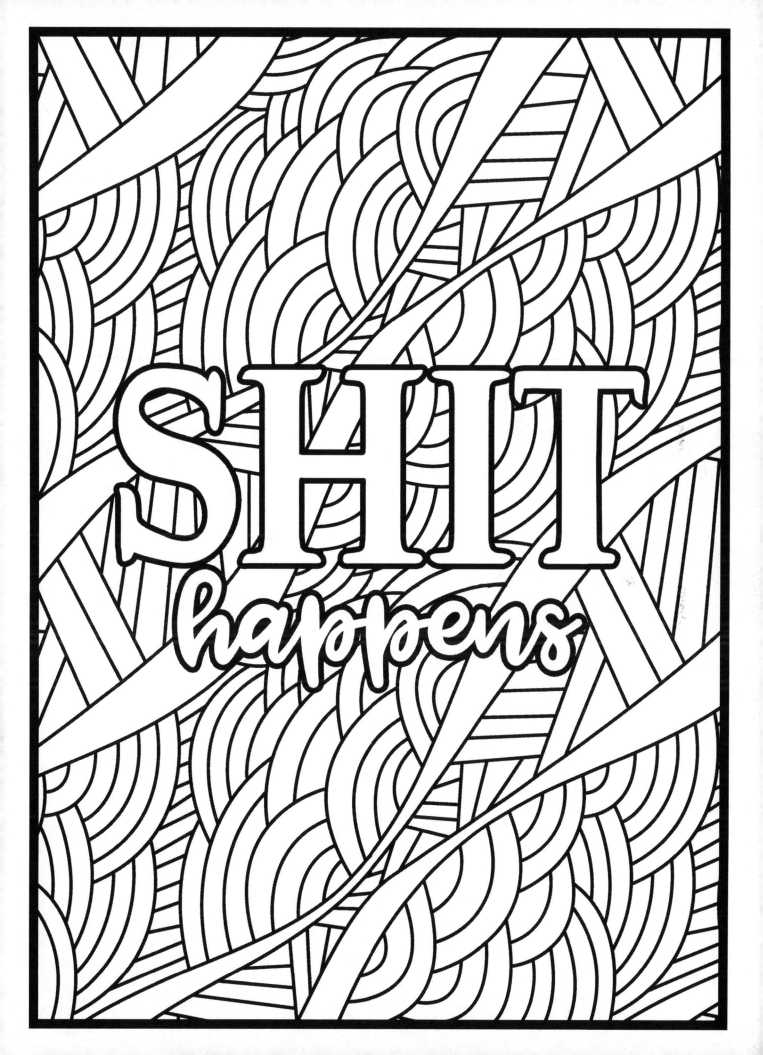

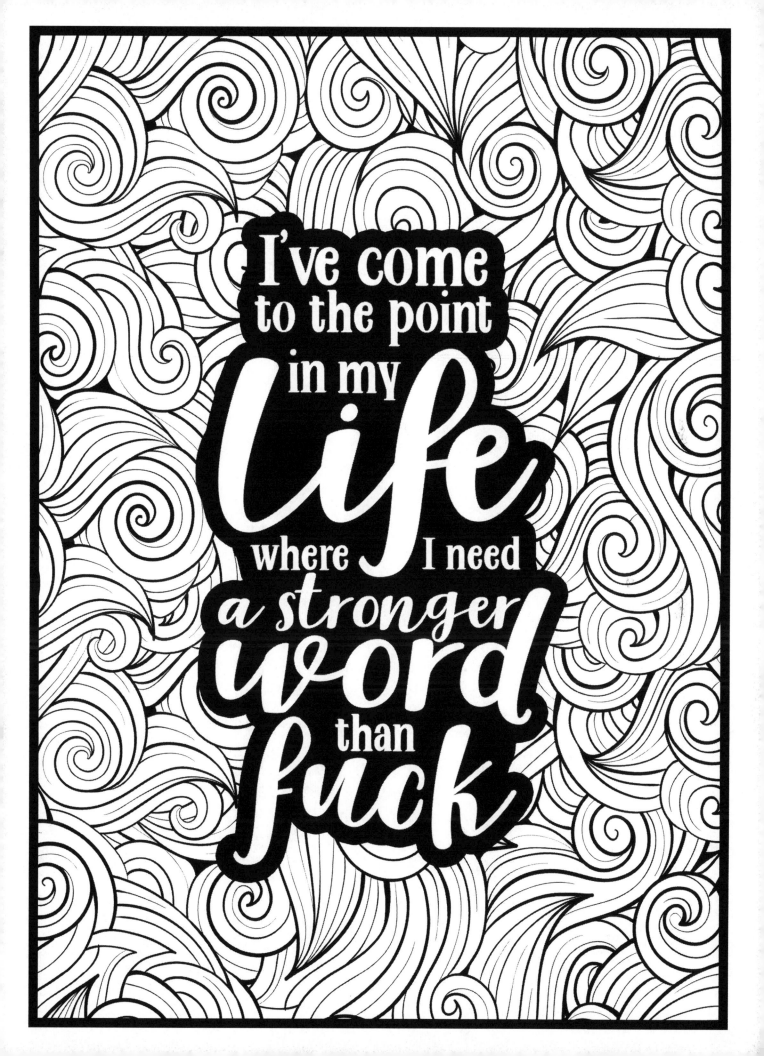

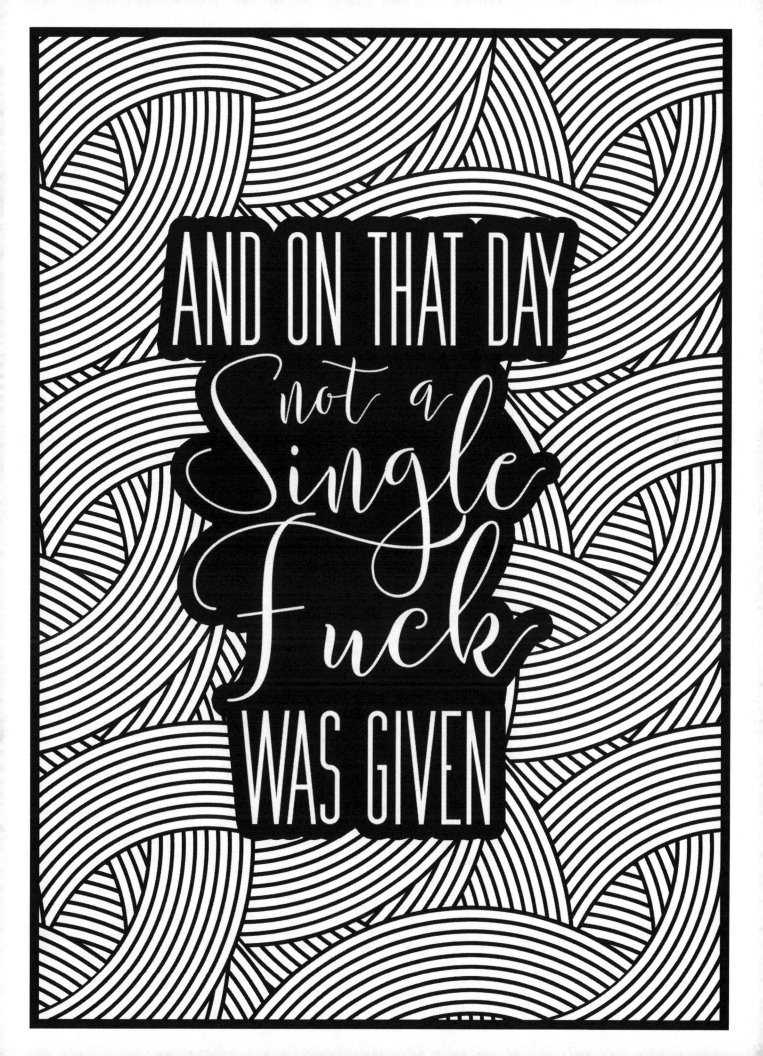

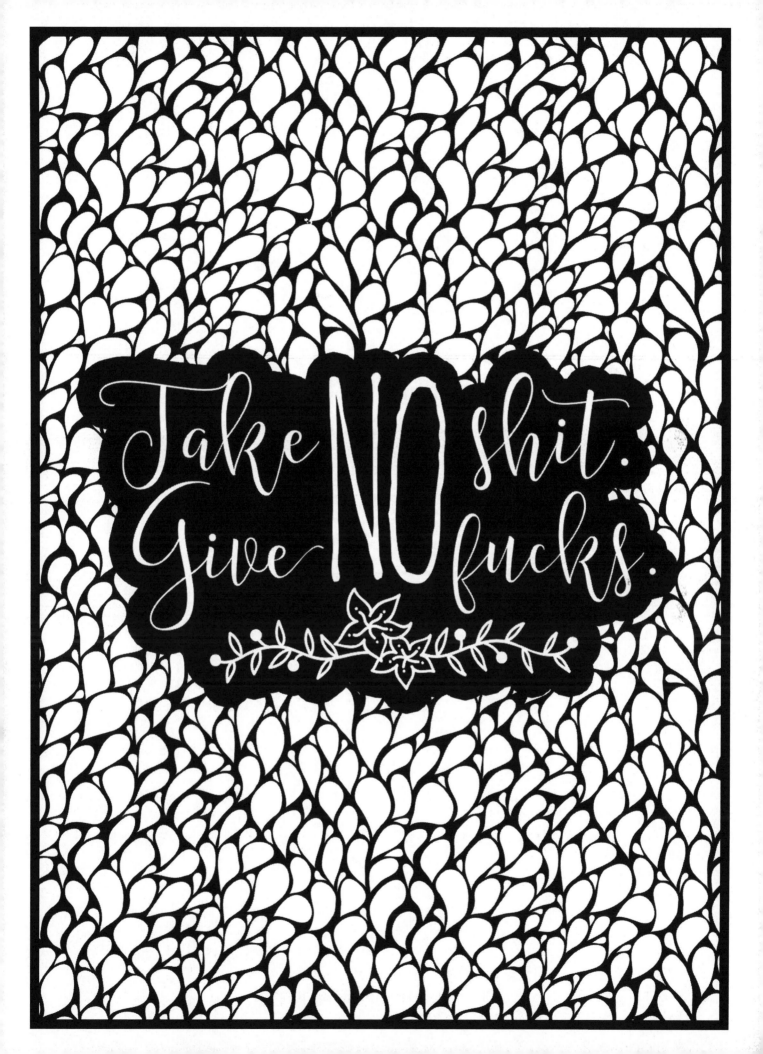

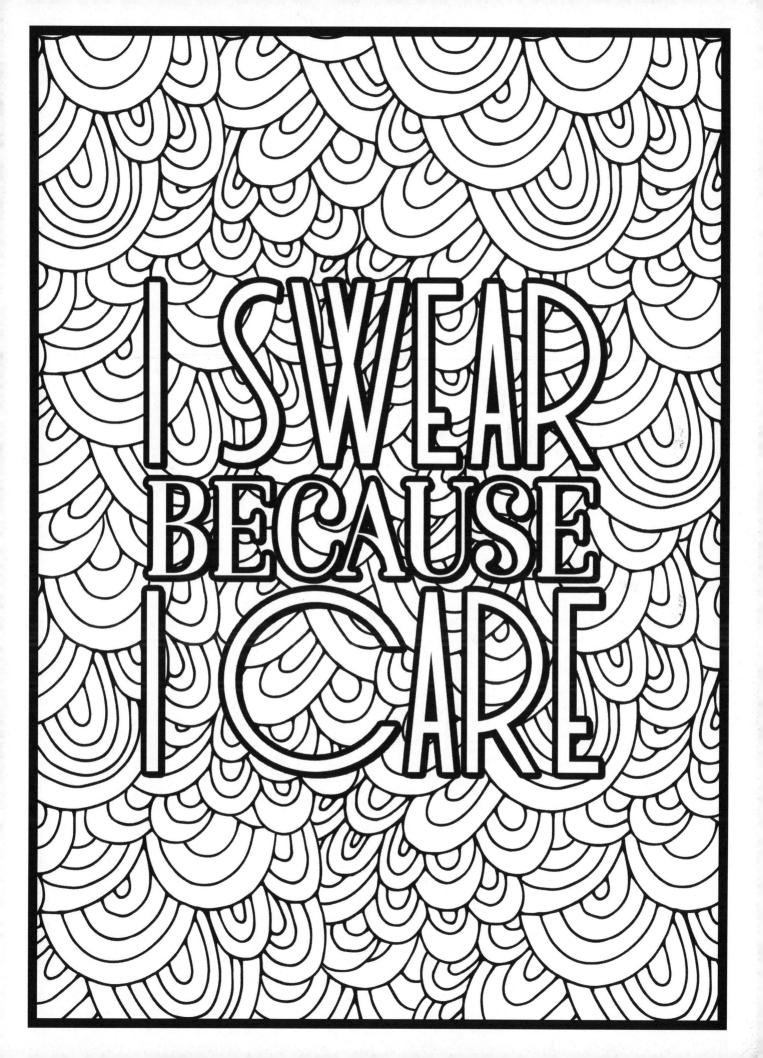

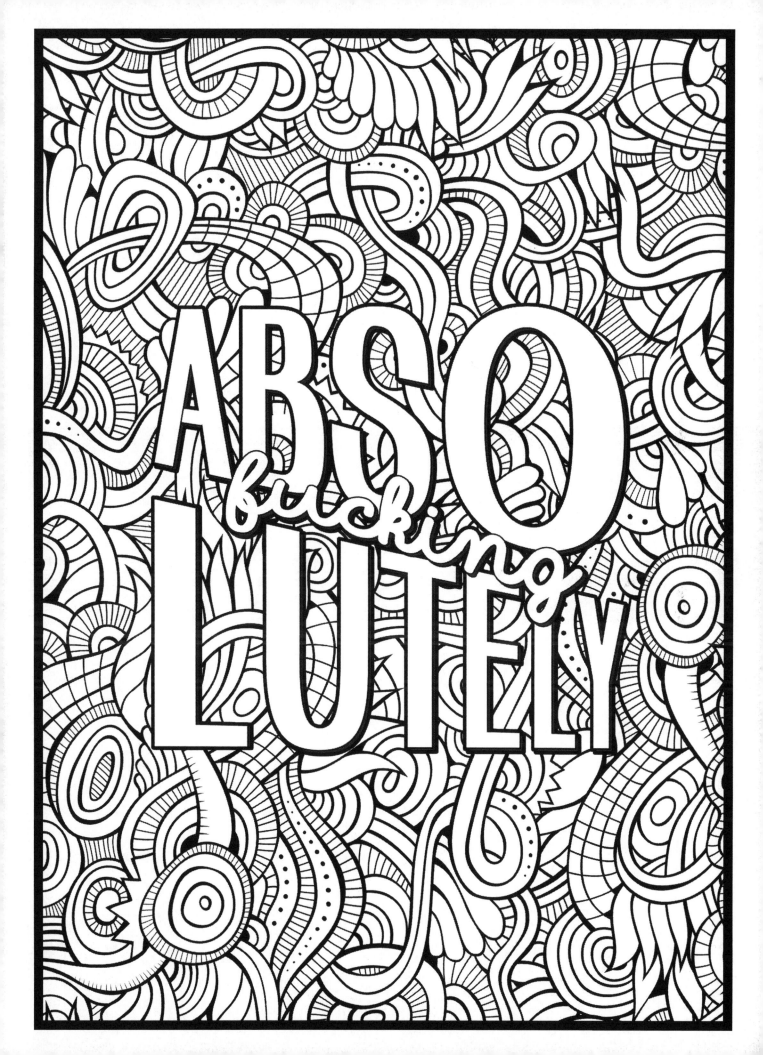

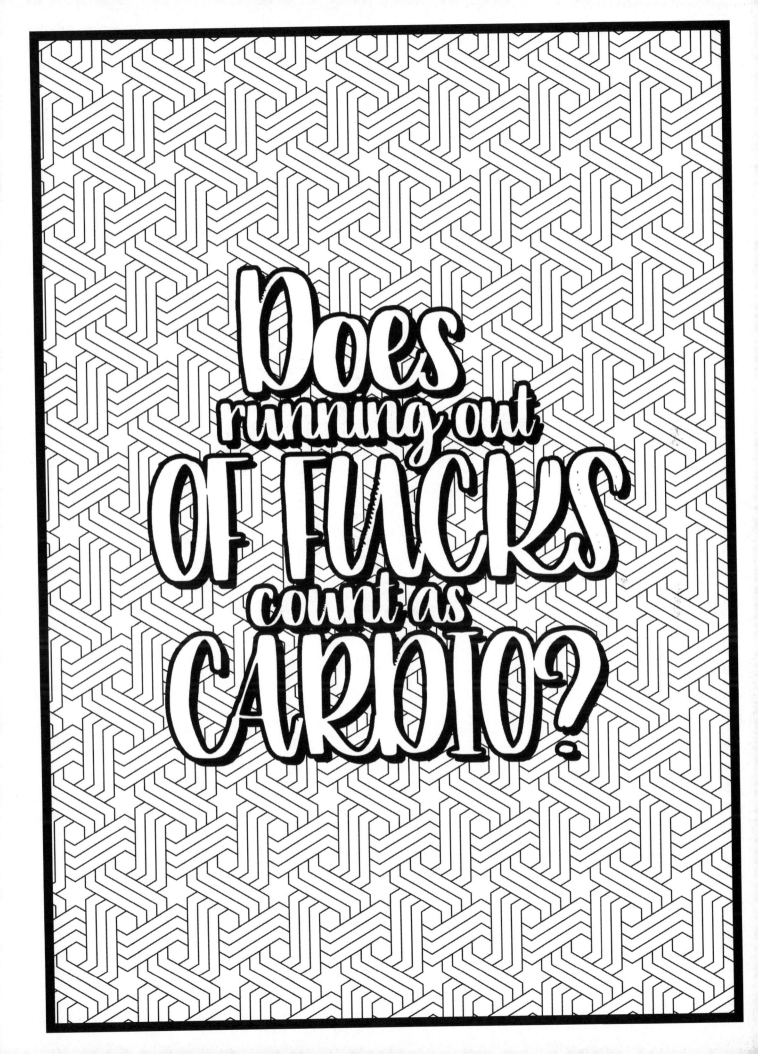

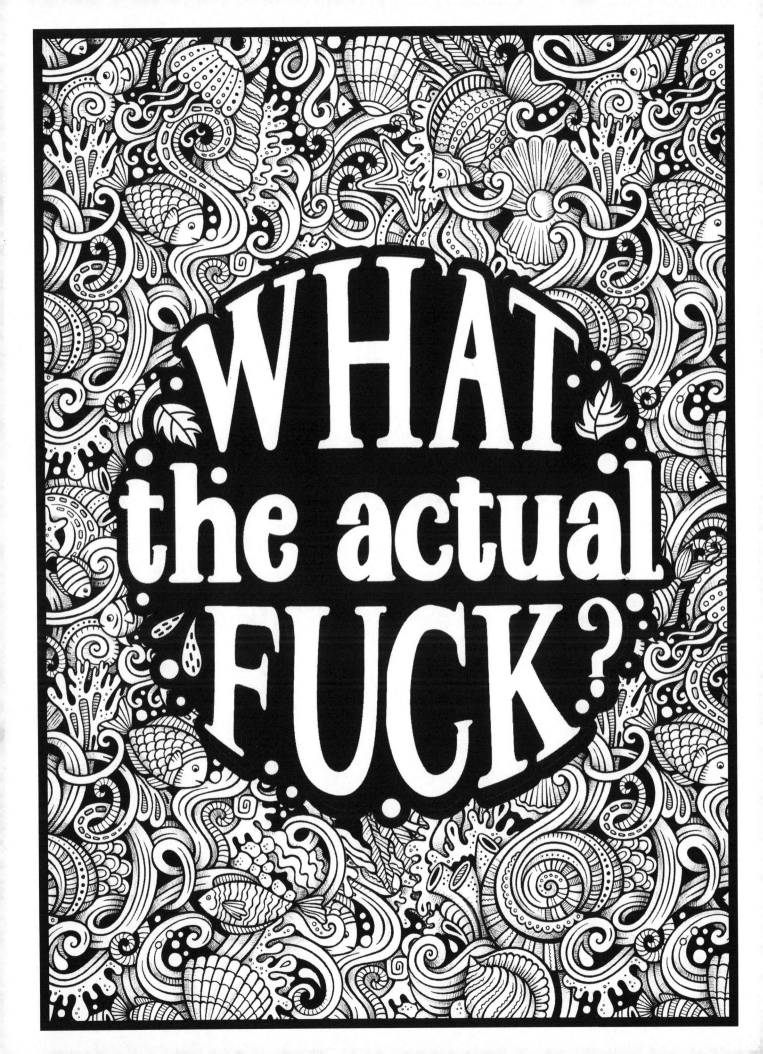

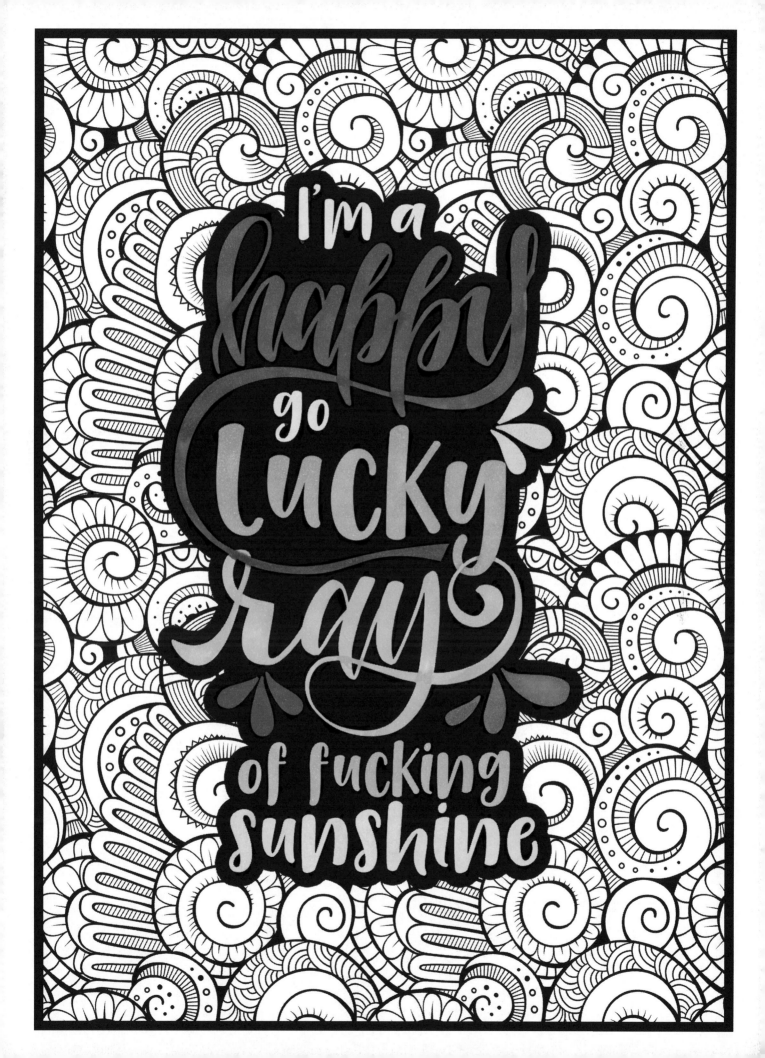

THE **I like** SOUND
you make when you
SHUT THE
FUCK UP

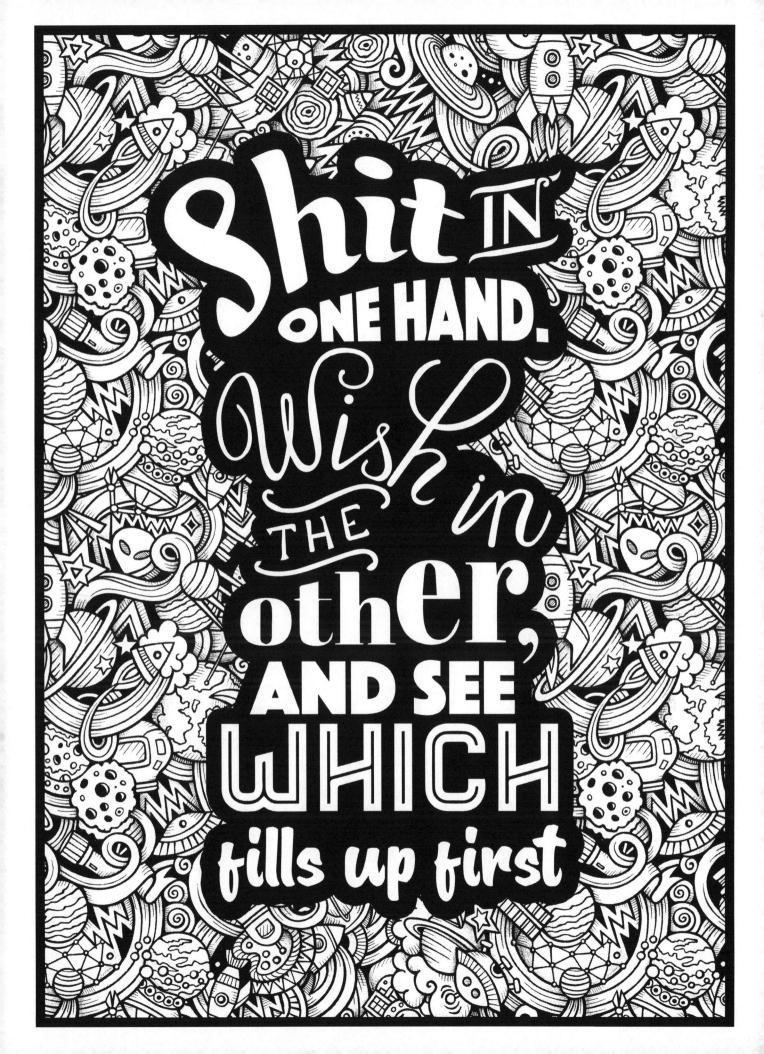

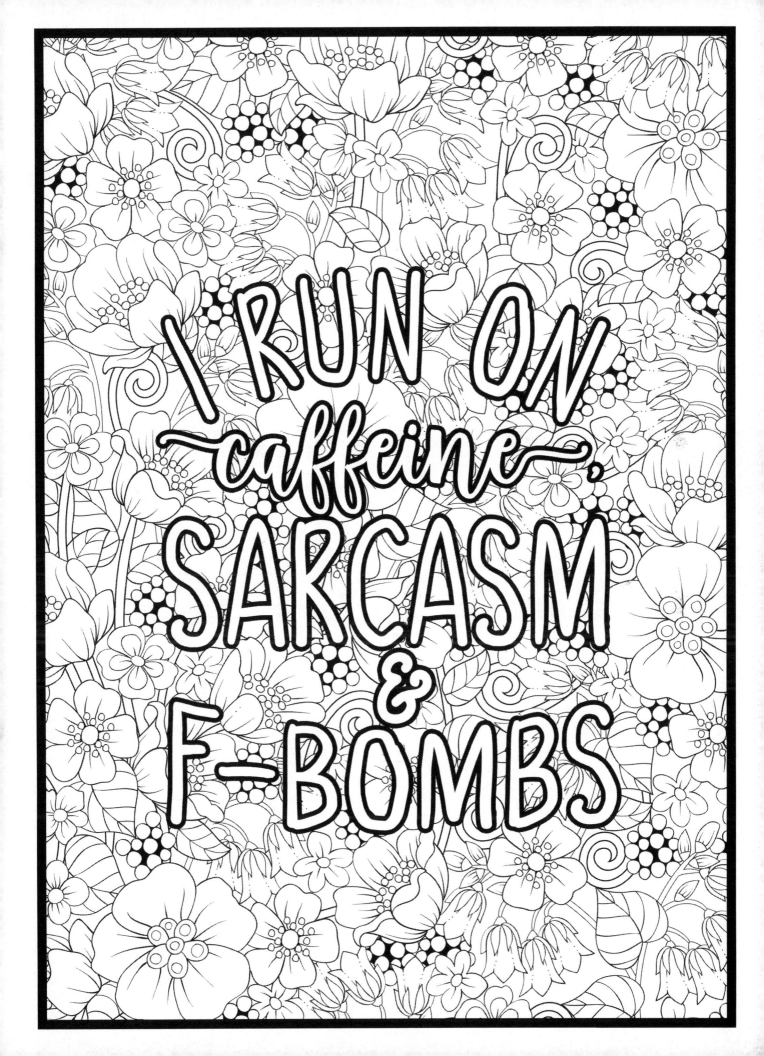

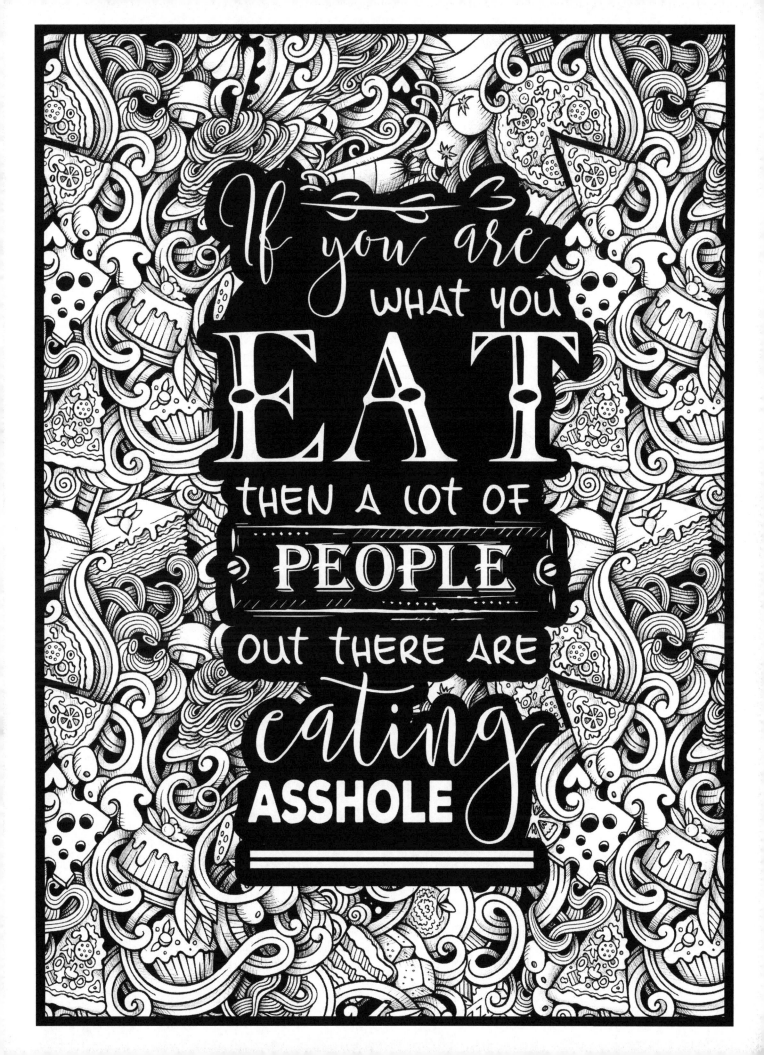

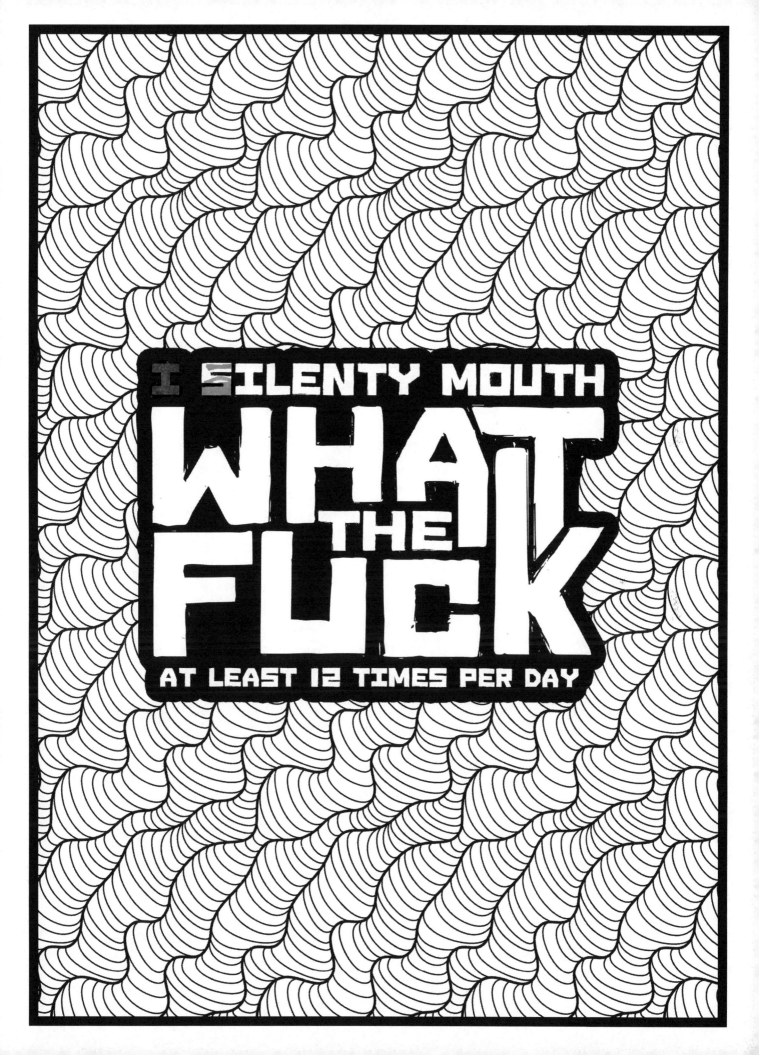

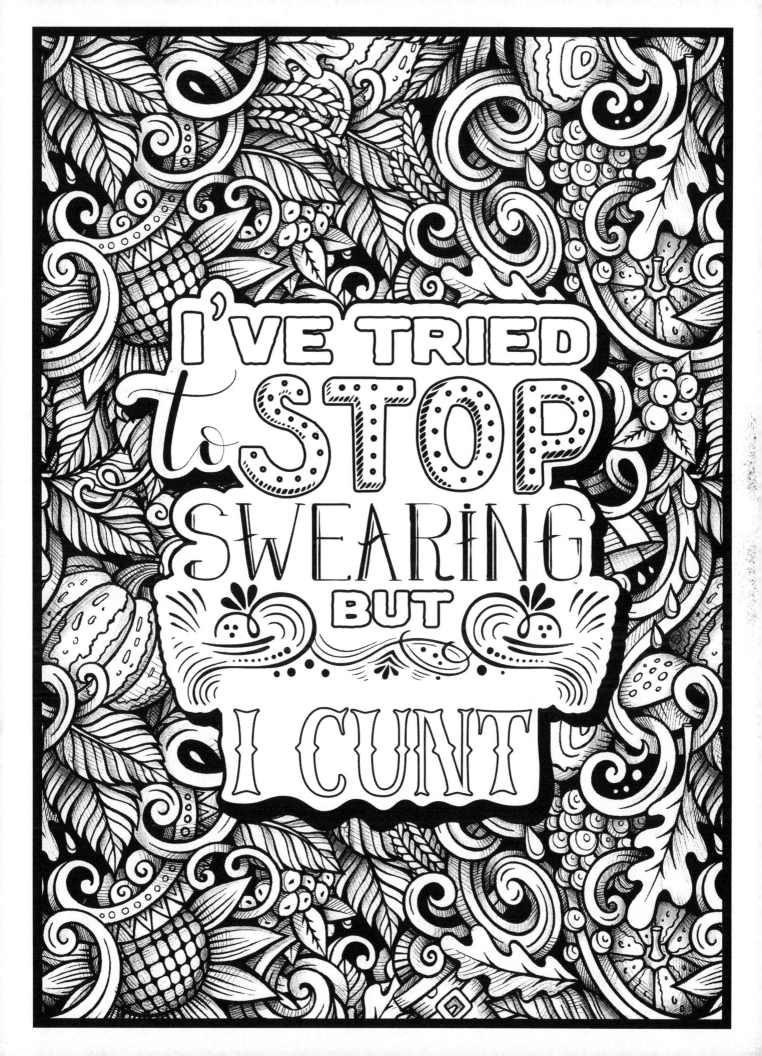

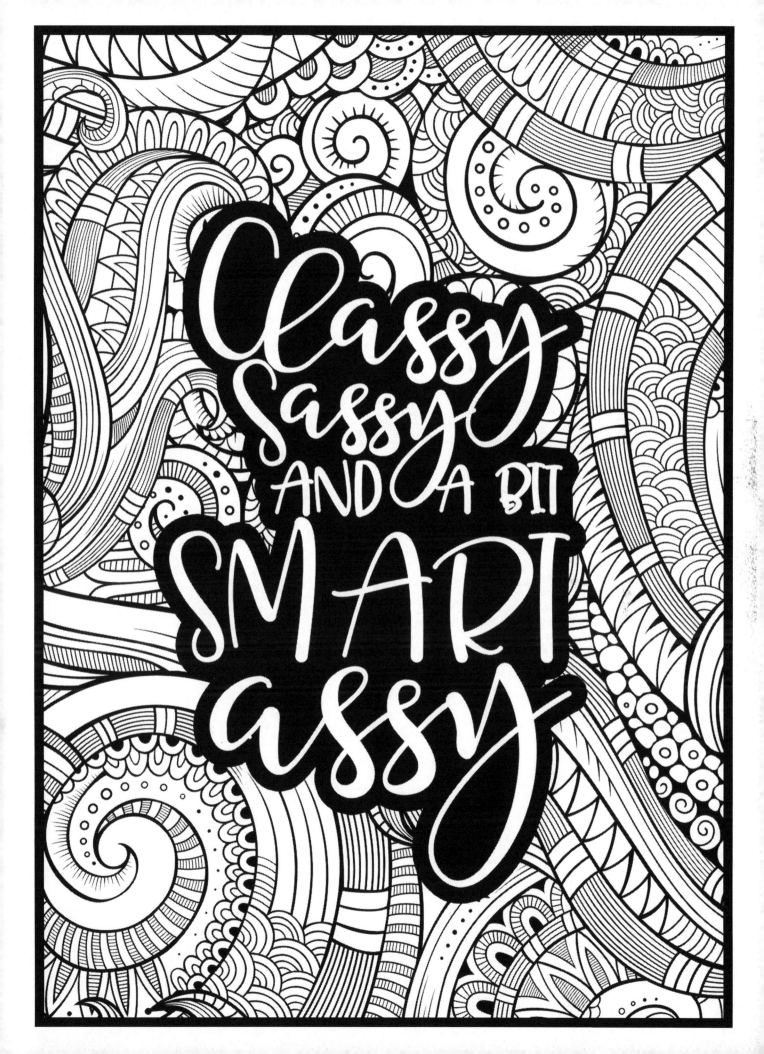

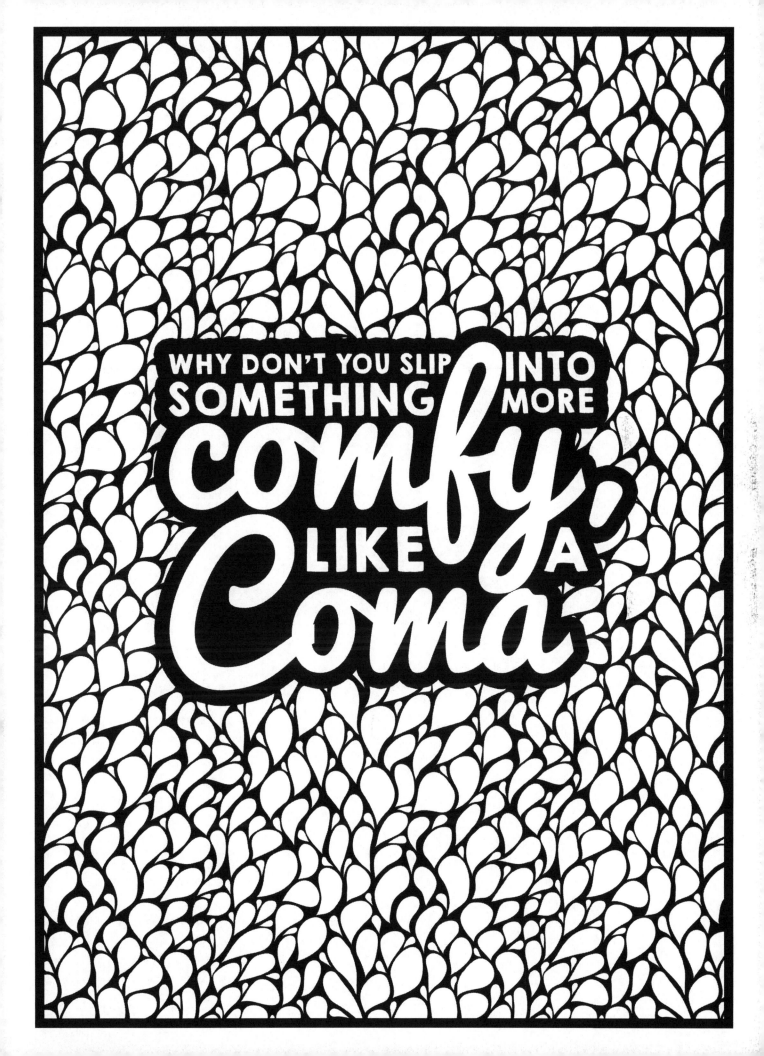

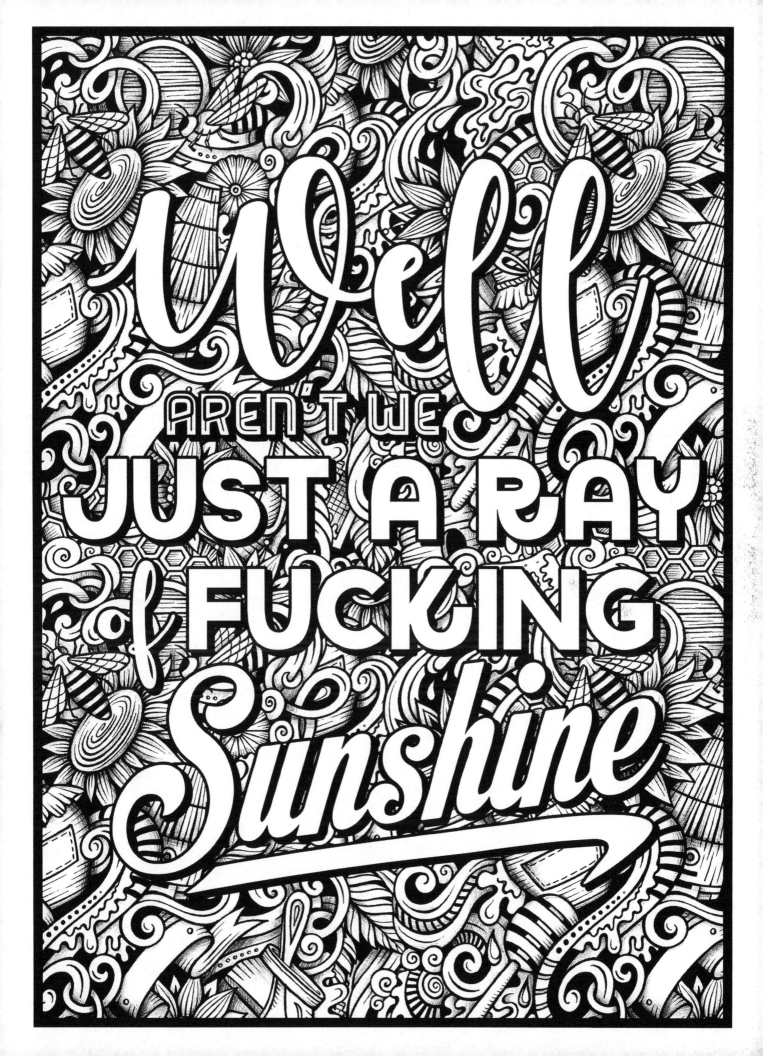

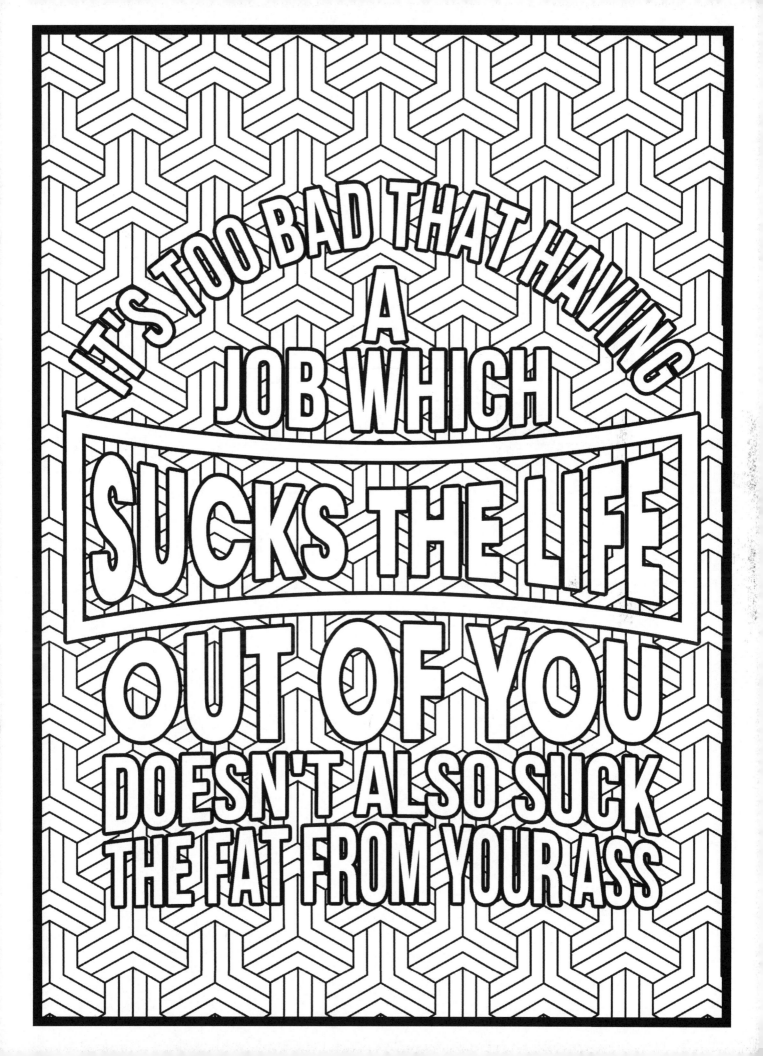

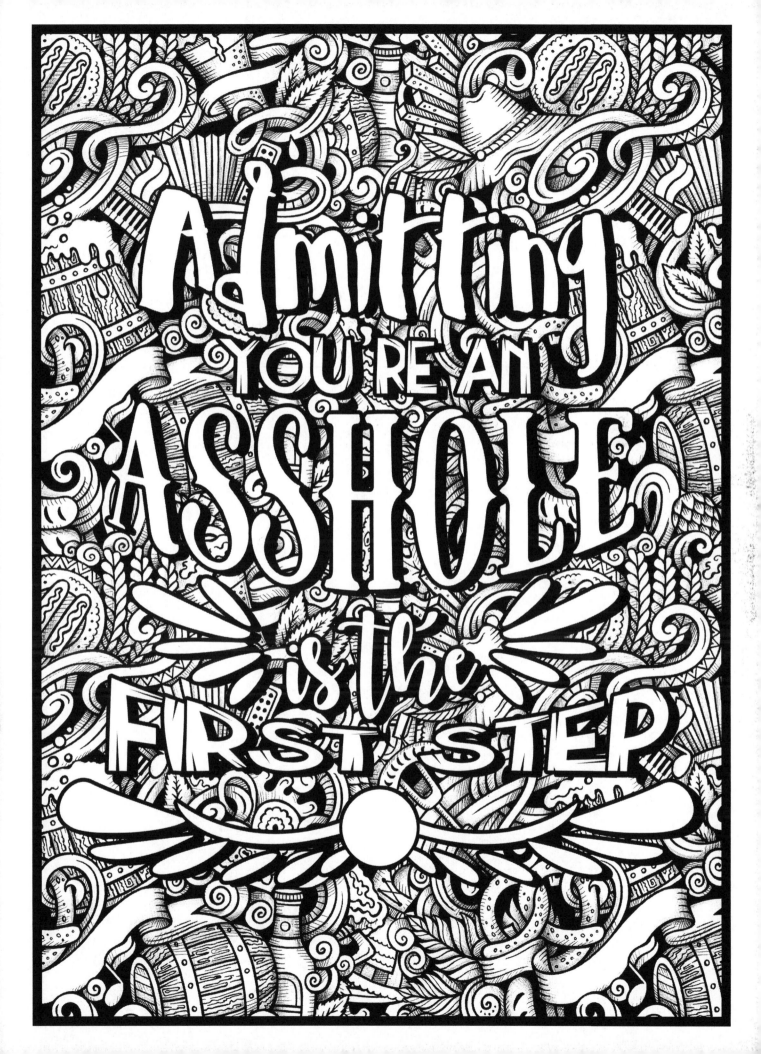

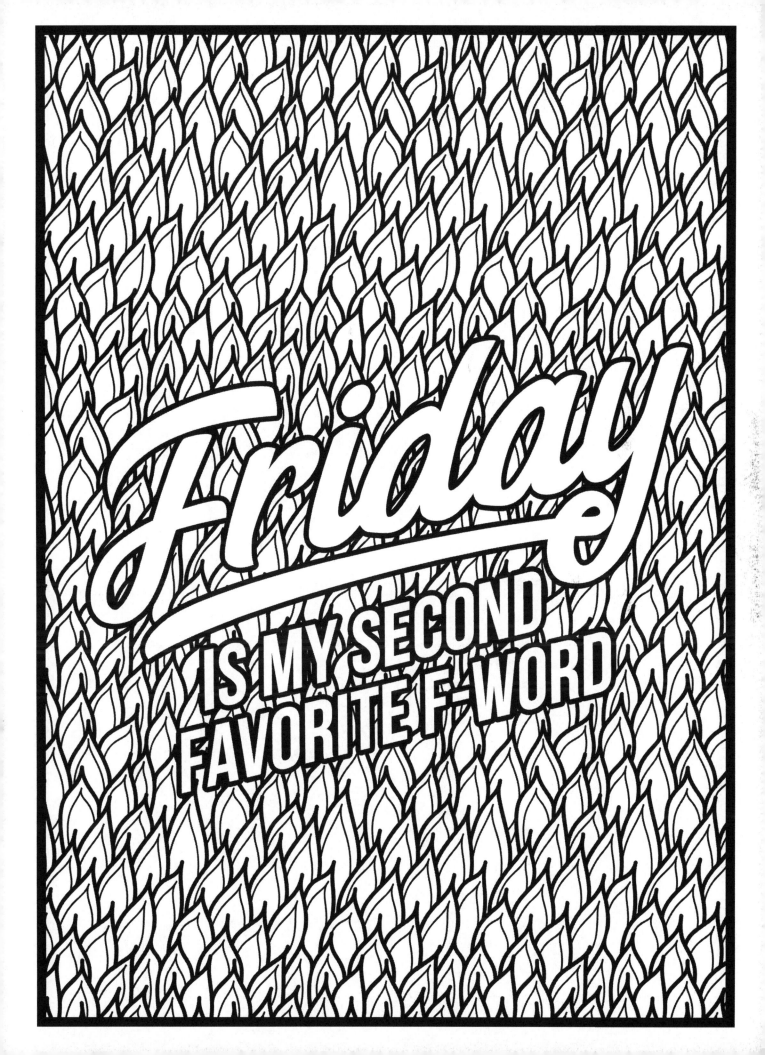

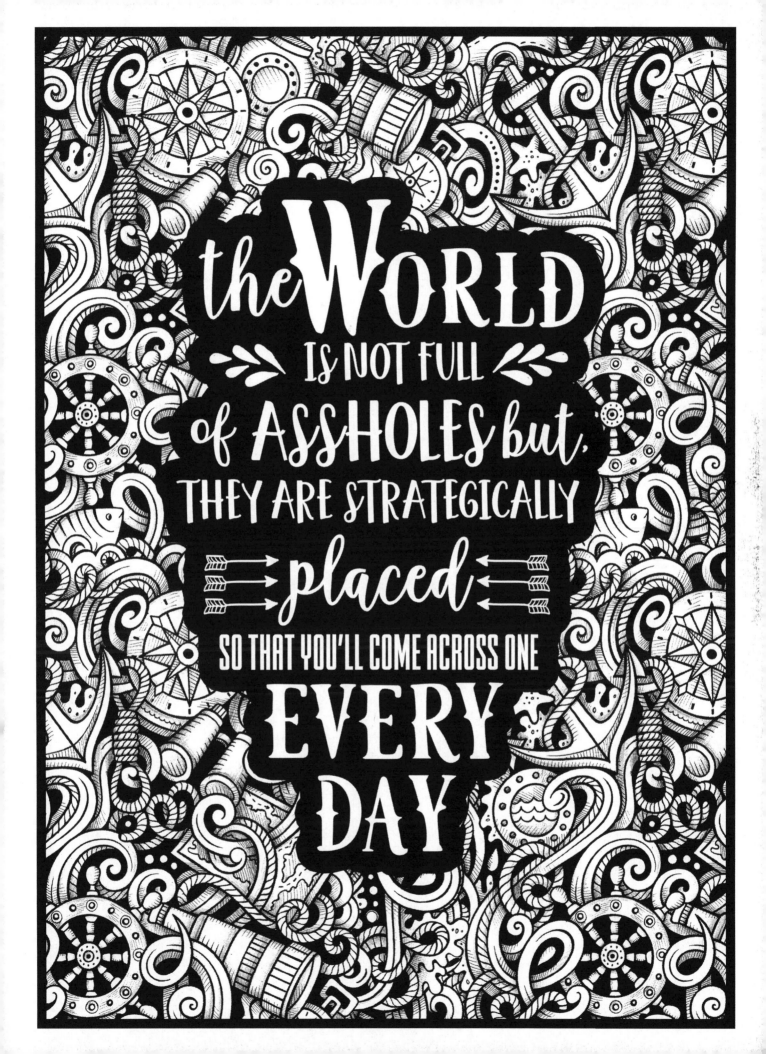

I am a nice PERSON. Just don't PUSH my BITCH button.

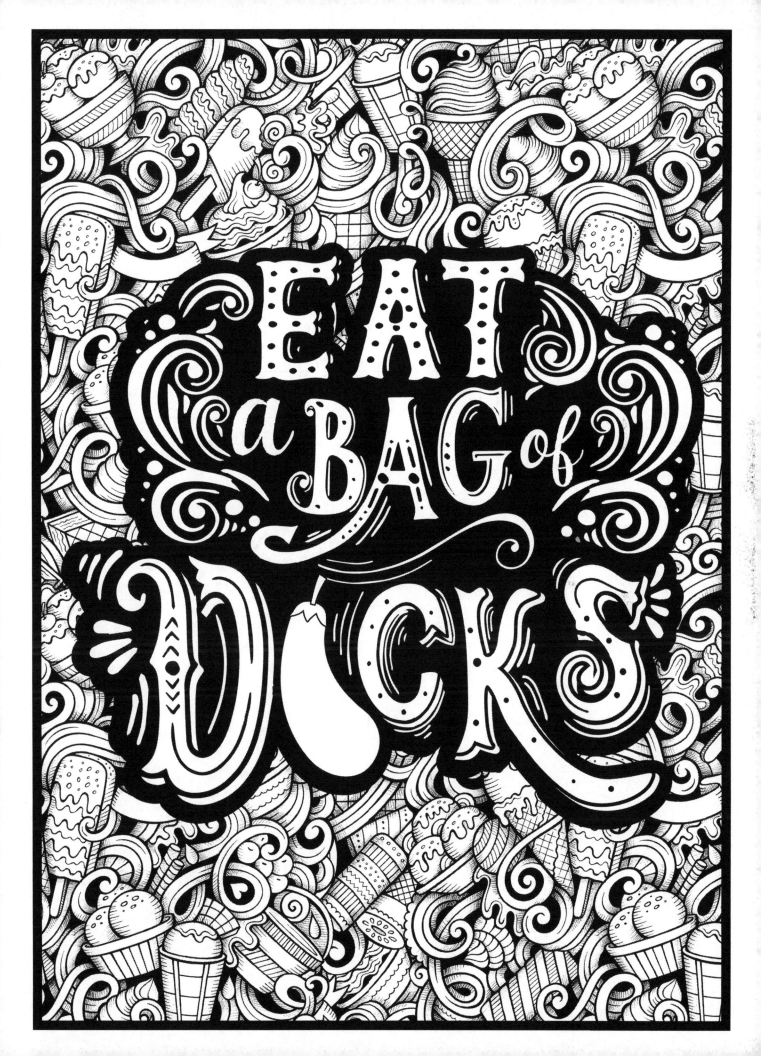

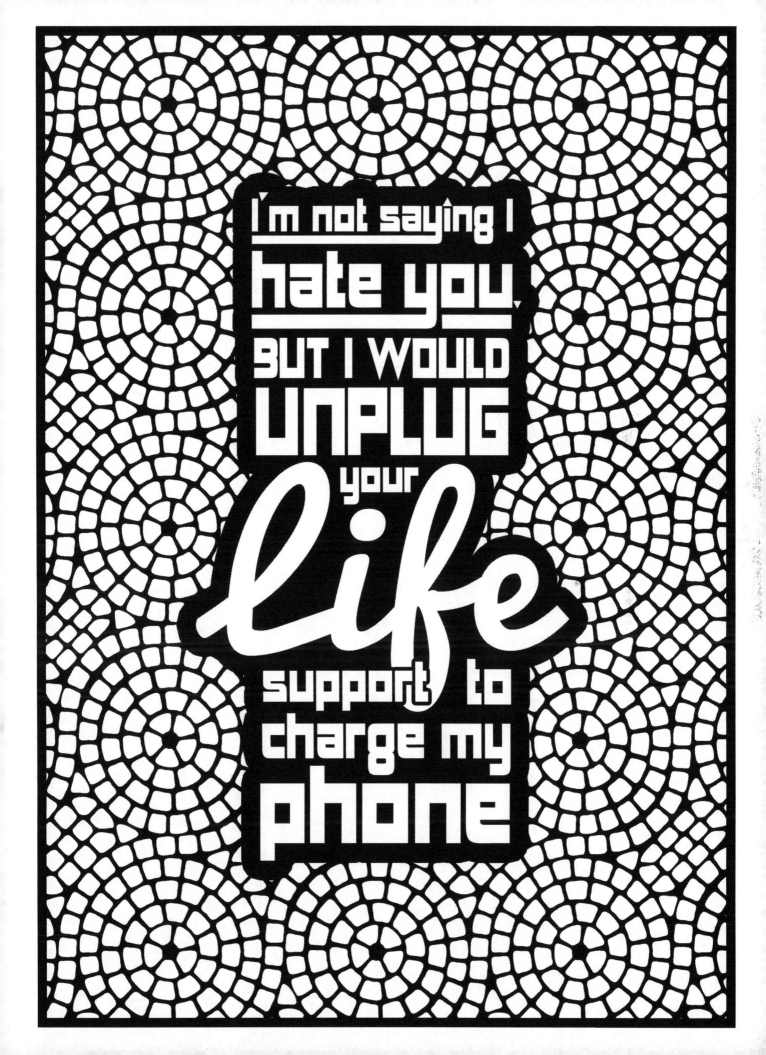

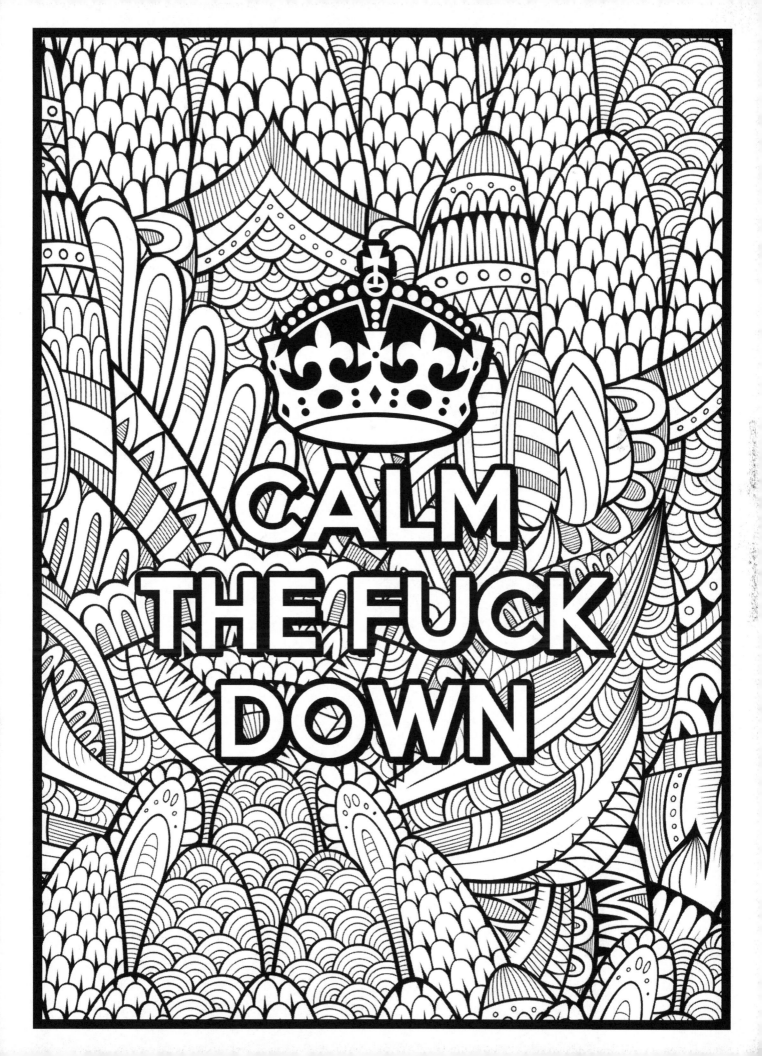

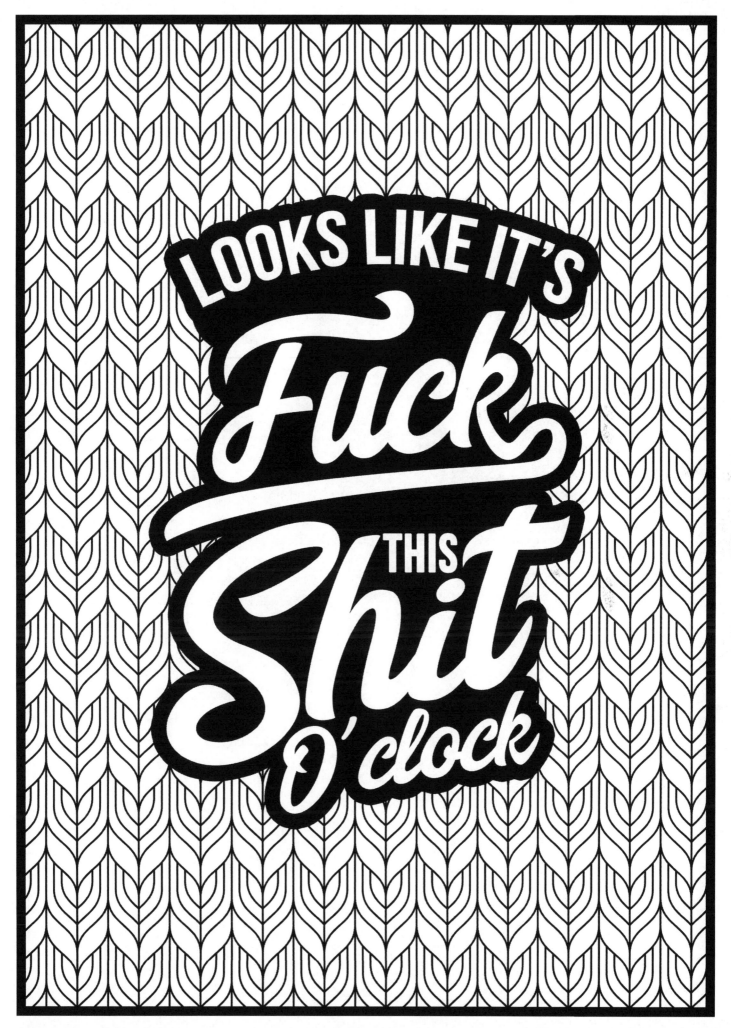

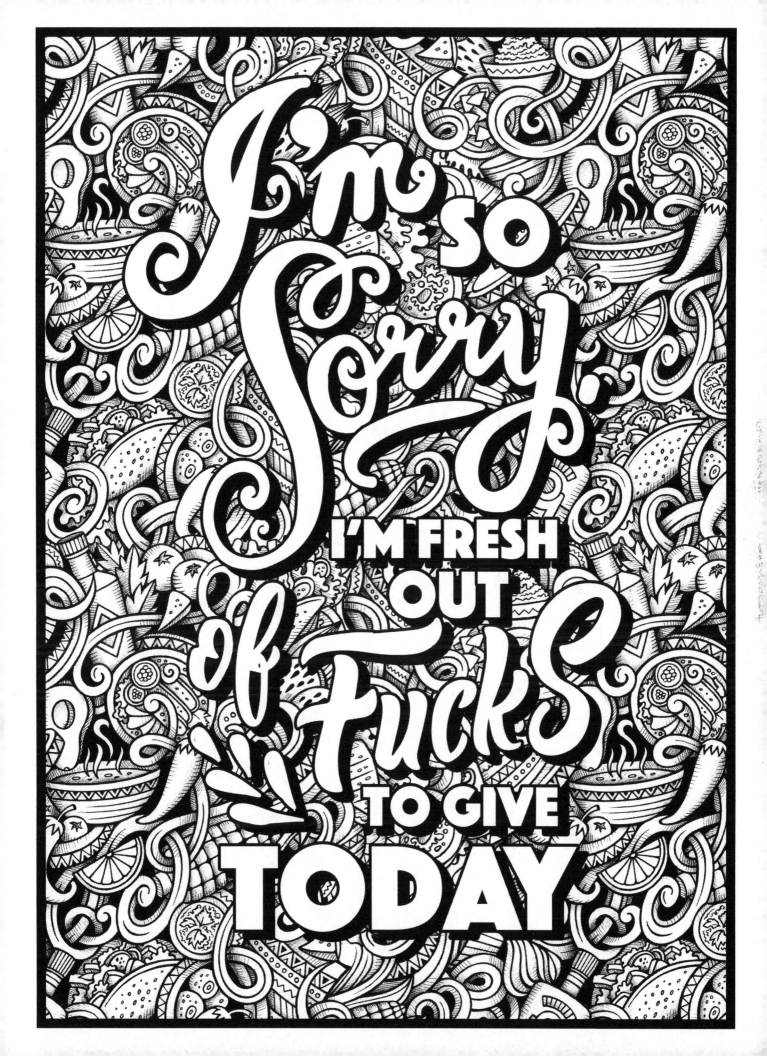

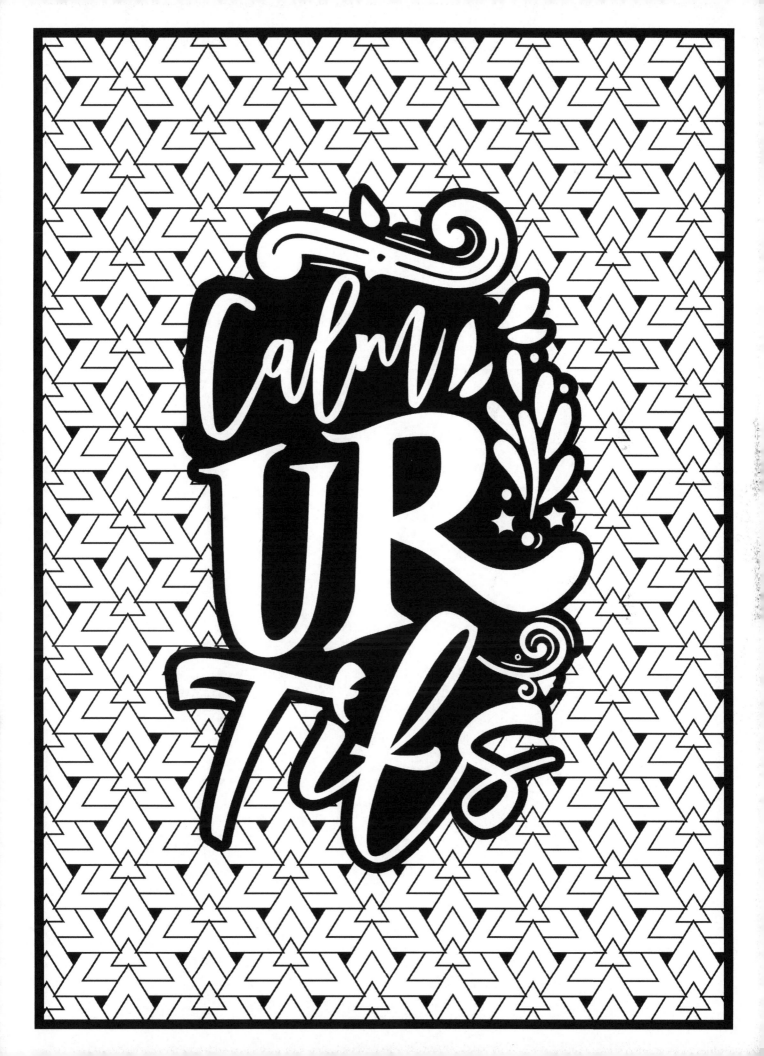

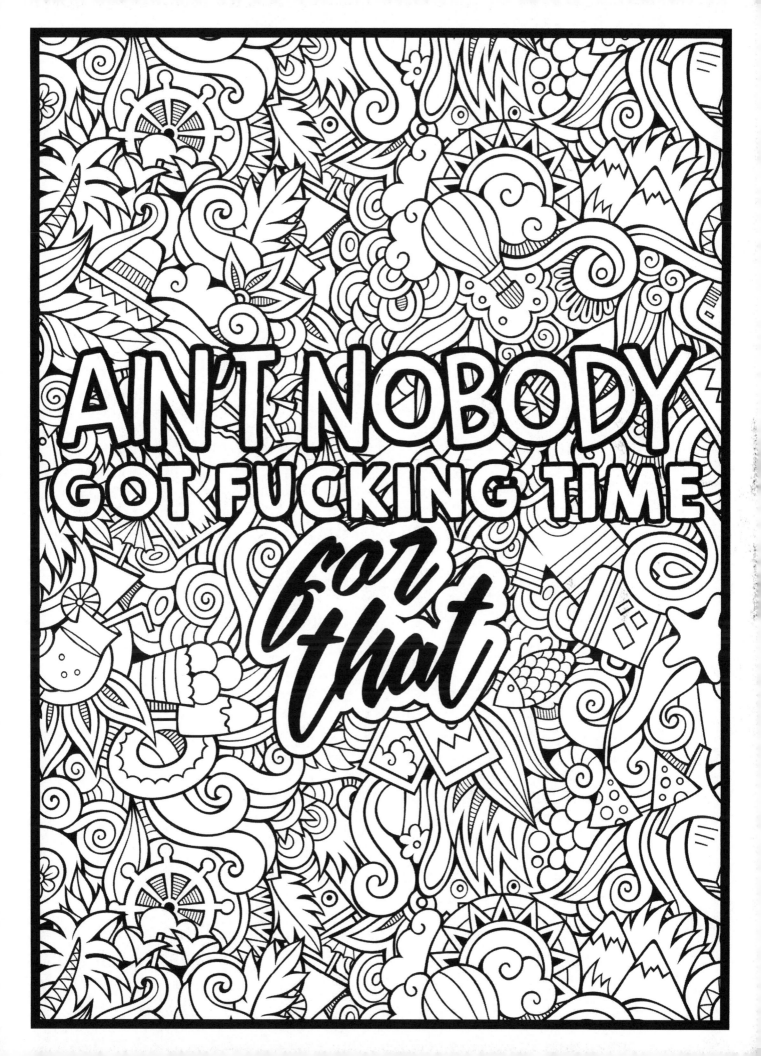

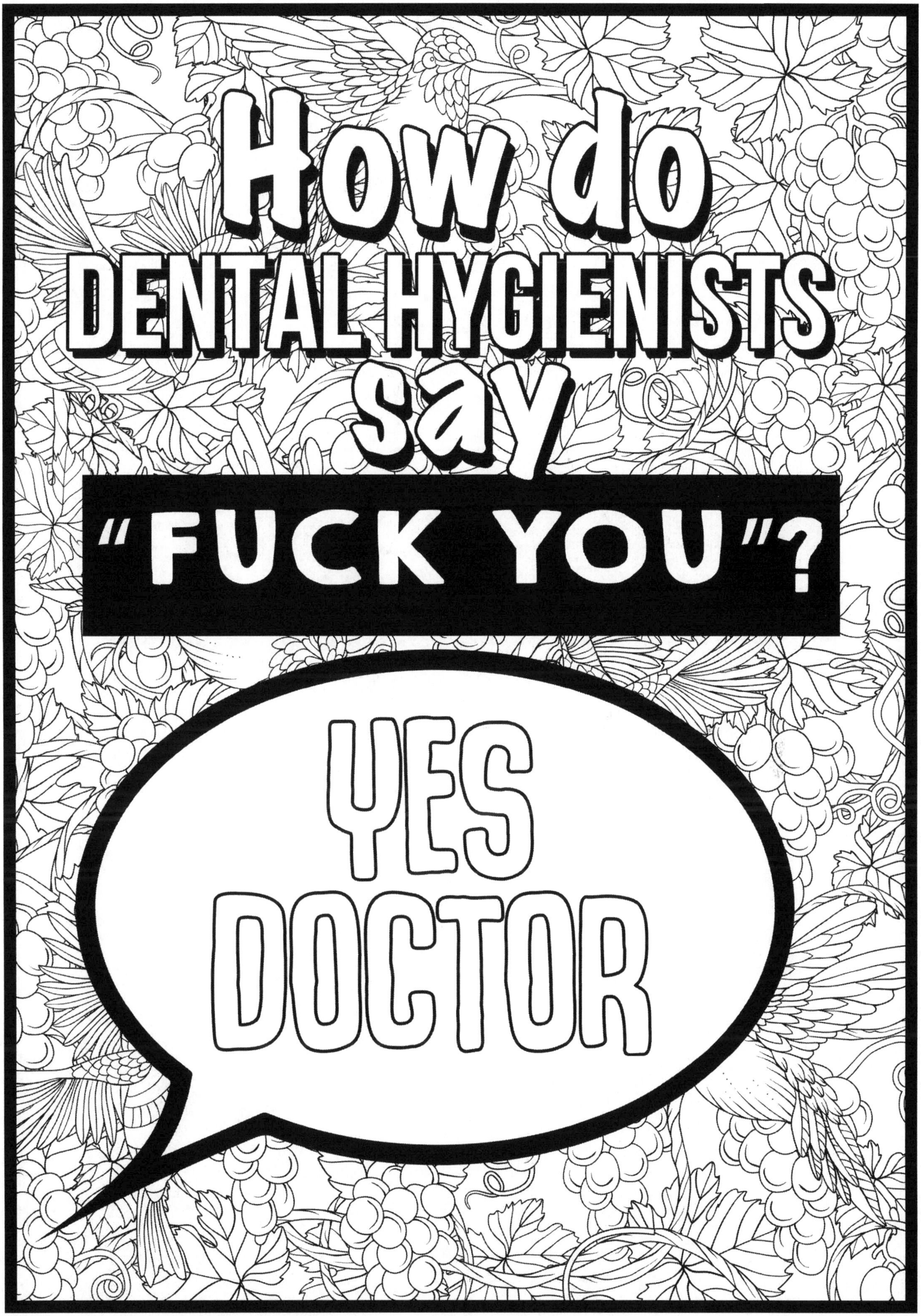
How do
DENTAL HYGIENISTS
say
"FUCK YOU"?
YES
DOCTOR

Want free goodies?
Email us at freebies@honeybadgercoloring.com

@honeybadgercoloring

Honey Badger Coloring

Shop our other books at
www.honeybadgercoloring.com

Wholesale distribution through Ingram Content Group
www.ingramcontent.com/publishers/distribution/wholesale

For questions and customer service, email us at
support@honeybadgercoloring.com

Made in the USA
Columbia, SC
12 December 2019